SKILLS AND LAW

MADE EASY

Tsong Yun Kwong is a medical graduate from Bart's and the London Medical School. He did an intercalated BSc at UCL and is currently undertaking his foundation training in London.

Qiang Kwong is a medical graduate from Oxford University. He did his pre-clinical studies at Cambridge University and is currently undertaking his foundation programme in London.

Ann O'Brien has been a practising GP for 28 years and, as such, values the benefits of effective and supportive communication with patients. She has been involved in undergraduate medical education for 15 years, both in practice and at Bart's and London School of Medicine and Dentistry. Her enthusiasm for imparting the skills of a good professional doctor and communicator has been the driving force in her participation in the editing of this book.

Joanne Haswell completed a Law degree at University College London, then qualified as a Barrister in 1998. Joanne has over 8 years' experience in developing training courses for healthcare professionals in the Law, has co-authored a web-based training programme on consent and has written numerous articles on Healthcare Law for both the national and specialist press.

Kate Hill is an Associate in the Healthcare team at RadcliffesLeBrasseur solicitors. During her career Kate has been involved in a number of high profile cases acting for the NHS. Two of her particular interests are informed consent and mental health. Kate has advised government organisations on the application of human rights legislation and has written practical protocols on the subject for other institutions. She is often consulted by Mental Health Trusts, including Special Hospitals.

For Elsevier:
Commissioning Editor: Timothy Horne
Development Editor: Sheila Black
Project Manager: Jane Dingwall
Designer: Charles Gray

MEDICAL COMMUNICATION SKILLS AND LAW

The Patient Centred Approach

MADE EASY

Tsong Yun Kwong BSc MBBS(London)
FY2 Doctor, Homerton NHS Trust, London, UK

Qiang Kwong MA(Cantab) BM BChir(Oxon)
FY2 Doctor, St Mary's Hospital NHS Trust, London, UK

Ann O'Brien MBBS(London) FRCGP DRCOG
Clinical Teaching Fellow, Academic Unit for Community Based Medical Education, Institute of
Health Sciences Education, Barts & London School of Medicine & Dentistry, London, UK

Joanne Haswell LLB(Hons)
Barrister; Director, InPractice Training, London, UK

Kate Hill BA(Hons)
Solicitor, RadcliffesLeBrasseur; Managing Director, InPractice Training, London, UK

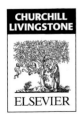

CHURCHILL LIVINGSTONE

ELSEVIER

Edinburgh London New York Oxford Philadelphia St Louis Sydney Toronto 2009

CHURCHILL
LIVINGSTONE
ELSEVIER

An imprint of Elsevier Limited

First published 2009

ISBN: 978-0-7020-3083-3

British Library Cataloguing in Publication Data
A catalogue record for this book is available from the British Library

Library of Congress Cataloging in Publication Data
A catalog record for this book is available from the Library of Congress

Notice
Neither the Publisher nor the Authors assume any responsibility for any loss or
injury and/or damage to persons or property arising out of or related to any use of
the material contained in this book. It is the responsibility of the treating practitioner,
relying on independent expertise and knowledge of the patient, to determine the
best treatment and method of application for the patient.

The Publisher

Printed in China

CONTENTS

6. Explaining drug Y

7. Explaining device Z

8. Explaining procedures

9. Explaining surgical operations

10. OSCE scenarios

ACKNOWLEDGEMENTS

The authors are grateful for advice provided by Paul Reid LLB(Hons) DipLP, Medical Litigation Team, Shepherd and Wedderburn, Glasgow, UK.

PREFACE

This book aims to fill a gap in the area of medical communication skills and the law. Current communication skills books are too descriptive, often with no leading conclusions on how to approach patients in the real world. With communication skills an ever increasing part of modern medical curricula, this lack of direction from books may make it difficult for those with poorer natural skills to improve in accordance with GMC directives.

This book's medical text is aimed at medical students of all years, junior doctors and those preparing for PLAB. It is designed to provide a basis for good clinical practice, but will also help the student pass their crucial exams and encourage the development of their own individual style.

From the authors' own experience, we know that prescriptive books can often be the best teaching tools. We wrote this book because we wanted to teach doctors about the information that *patients* want, delivered in a manner to provide the best outcome for all.

We feel that this is the first book to give medical students, as well as overseas and junior doctors, detailed tools to explain test results, diseases, drugs, devices, procedures and operations, in the way patients want. We have given our material to our own patients for comment and have been given the stamp of approval by them.

For each of the common areas required when treating patients, we have given examples. The information we give is a solid starting block on what to say and, perhaps, how to say it. In your own time you will of course develop your own style. We have also included examples of the most common diseases, drugs and devices. We hope this might save the reader time when revising for exams.

Legal books often suffer from the same problem as communication skills books and so we have given the legal sections the same treatment. We have made them similarly prescriptive and included the most up-to-date material from healthcare lawyers at a leading solicitors firm (RadcliffesLeBrasseur) and medico-legal training company (InPractice).

Finally, we have combined the legal sections with the relevant communication skills to add relevance to the material. These legal sections, under the *Legal Guidance* headings, integrate the legal basis of medicine with helpful advice, in an attempt to minimise the risk of complaints and proceedings. We feel that some applied understanding of the common legal areas for medics will assist in your daily practice. Some practice notes have been included, as well as some of the more common medico-legal pitfalls to be avoided.

May this book give you exam success!!!

London 2009

Tsong Yun Kwong
Qiang Kwong
Ann O'Brien
Joanne Haswell
Kate Hill

The basics

INTRODUCTION

All patients want a good relationship with their doctors. It should be a relationship of honesty, openness and privacy. However, achieving this ideal is hard because of the many complex factors involved.

The current trend is to move away from the paternalistic approach towards a cooperative approach between the health expert and the patient, where the doctor gives the patient all the facts about possible courses of action and it is the patient who decides which course of action is best for them.

Rapport

Simply put, rapport is how well a doctor and patient get on, and it is the **most** important aspect of doctor–patient communication. If we like someone, then we are more likely to respect them and value their opinion. If your patient likes and respects you, he is more likely to adhere to treatment, and so on. For patients within a GP practice, rapport with their physician is the most important factor affecting whether patients follow the physician's advice or not.

How to improve the rapport with a patient:

- Appearance: smart dress; proper ID showing.
- Good, clear introduction (the need to develop a good first impression).
- Language: lack of medical terms, minimal slang and no swearing.
- Approach: friendly, open, non-judgemental, accepting patients for who they are, interested in what the patient is saying and seen to be actively taking it in.
- Be appropriately reassuring and give words of encouragement.
- Develop a human side and become personable, possibly include personal tales/anecdotes.

After building rapport, the next major challenge is to develop professional techniques for dealing with patients in all kinds of scenarios, from figuring out diagnoses to delivering bad news or explaining new medication.

THE BASICS OF MEDICAL INTERACTION

In any clinical interaction, there are several key factors that determine its success. They are:

- the setting
- how to introduce yourself
- the questions asked
- the questions answered
- conduct when not speaking
- finishing off the interview.

The setting

Consider the three Ws:

- Where – clinic rooms versus bedside.
- Who should be present? (relatives/doctors/translator/ advocate services).
- When – a dedicated slot of time versus an incidental gap between jobs (be aware that time required may be more than you think).

How to introduce yourself

A tried and tested method is as follows:

- Introductory greeting – *hi, hello, good morning.*
- Find out how the patient wants to be known, e.g. Mr Smith, Brian, Dr Brown.
- Say who you are, your name and who you represent, e.g. *I'm Dr Smith from the surgical team/emergency cover/ heart team, etc. I work with the consultant Dr Jones.*

- Explain why you are there and obtain consent – *I've been asked to review you by colleagues because of the pain you're experiencing. Is it okay if I ask you some questions and examine you? I will share the information you give me with my colleagues.*
- Establish the level of understanding – make sure the patient understands where you fit into the team and at what level you are clinically responsible.
- By using a leading phrase, you can encourage the patient to start explaining their problems:
  - *What seems to be the matter/problem?*
  - *What has brought you into the clinic/A+E today?*
  - *Would you please tell me what has been happening to you?*

The use of jargon can result in the patient not understanding the information. This lack of understanding vitiates (invalidates) consent and any subsequent consent will be unlawful.

Be careful not to overstep the mark with personal tales. In particular, do not use overly persuasive phrases such as – *I would tell my own mother to do this.*

How to ask questions

- Questions should initially be **open**, e.g. *Tell me what's been going on. What can I do to help?* Then listen.
- If questions need to be asked to exclude important factors, they should be specific to the information needed.
- If difficult questions need to be asked, then these can be **signposted**, i.e. given forewarning, so the question is less likely to surprise, e.g. *Your problem seems to be related to intimate areas, so I need to ask some questions that are very personal – questions regarding your sex life. Is that okay?*

- Clarify what a patient means. *I'm ill* – does that mean a headache/chest pain/earache?
- Use terms appropriate to different cultures.

It is a good idea to summarise any key points that the patient makes, e.g. the details of his/her chest pain, since the history is key to the diagnosis. You could also summarise if there is a difficult silence or when you've run out of questions at that point, e.g. *Mrs X, you were telling me that your chest pain came on this morning quite suddenly and that you were coughing up a little blood as well, but you weren't particularly short of breath, though...*, and this can lead to further information from the patient.

Answering questions

Patient's agenda

The patient's agenda is defined as those areas of a consultation which address the patient's intentions/expectations. Ask yourself if a patient has come with an anticipated outcome.

 Tip – If possible document the patient's expected outcome verbatim in the notes.

Why is the patient's agenda important? Understanding the patient's approach to the consultation means that you can adapt your style to work with the patient to reach the best outcome for them.

You should consider:

- the patient's emotions – fearfulness/apprehension/ concern over their own health or that of others
- the origins of the patient's health beliefs – patient's relatives' experiences and what they have read
- what patients want out of the consultation – equality of the position, expecting the truth or a prescription at the end.

Respond to patient cues

In order to answer a patient's questions and respond to their concerns, you have to look at how your patient's behaviour changes during the interaction. This may range from a subtle change in the emphasis of words to obvious emotional outpourings or to changes in posture. It is impossible to list the possible meanings of a patient's body language. However, some are common, e.g.:

- Slowing down or increasing hesitancy suggests the patient is trying to digest information, so you should **slow** down, repeat and summarise, invite questions or break off.
- Silence can indicate that the patient is overwhelmed with information or emotion. They may not understand what is being said – give the patient time to assimilate the information (**wait**).

You should continuously monitor and check the understanding of the patient and how much information the patient can cope with. Make sure the patient can hear what is being said – communication can be hampered by background noise, if you have a soft voice or if the patient is hard of hearing.

What patients want to hear:

- truthful, honest answers
- what your line of thinking is at the moment
- information at a pace they can understand, so they're not left behind
- a measure of how serious a condition is and how the situation will immediately affect them
- appropriate reassurance
- medical jargon explained or avoided, using common layman's words to describe tests, e.g. say **heart attack** not **myocardial infarction**

- what happens to the average patient, e.g. prognosis, effects of drugs and relating it back to the patient on a personal level
- sparing use of statistics – some patients may prefer to hear the words **common** or **rare,** rather than percentages, or comparison to well-known events, e.g. winning the lottery/being knocked down by a car
- a plan for the way forward, without being dictatorial. A collaborative approach is found to be most effective.

Remember that there are limits to your own knowledge. If you cannot answer questions, offer to return with answers once you've consulted your seniors. Giving incorrect information is worse than providing none.

Conduct when not speaking

Empathy

I'm in pain may be one of the most common complaints heard by a doctor, but if the doctor has no personal experience of the type of pain complained of, they will never really truly understand it. However, that does not mean that doctors cannot show an appreciation of the suffering involved. Good patient care demands some level of understanding to build a successful connection. Empathy will come from efforts to get this right.

Simple phrases and actions during the conversation can greatly benefit the conversation. These include:

- looking concerned and interested in what the patient is saying by showing positive body language (see below) – this can be regarded as **active listening**
- genuinely meaning it when you are saying – *that must be hard/difficult for you*, or *I can understand the stress you were under*

- giving the patient time to express themselves and not rushing into giving solutions, which they may not be looking for.

Positive body language

- Eye contact.
- Nodding and agreeing (saying *uh-huh*), which shows that you arc taking an active interest.
- Looking the patient in the eye and facing them while they're talking (avoid putting your head down in the notes or typing on a computer).
- Not fidgeting (e.g. doodling on a piece of paper).
- Sitting forward in the chair to show interest, without crowding the patient.

Finishing the consultation

In most interviews, there is a natural end point and, provided you are satisfied with the information gained, you can end the interview by:

- inviting questions
- summarising the history and most likely diagnosis
- summarising the management plan derived from the meeting.

End the consultation with – *Thank you very much for telling me about your current problem. If you have any further questions, then please don't hesitate to call me, my colleague or any of the nursing staff.*

Other ways of improving communication

As well as developing good technique for communicating with body language and appropriate spoken language, there are other ways to improve communication:

- Updating documentation immediately after a

consultation (write down time/date, who was present, summary and your name/grade/bleep number)
- Being prepared to negotiate treatment and management plans with the patient
- Drawings and sketches
- Writing key words down for the patient to take away, e.g. conditions and drug names and treatment regimes
- Information leaflets
- Website addresses
- Support group contact details
- Summary letters to the patient after the consultation
- Referral to specialist nurses
- Patient advocates
- Suggest they get a friend or relative to support them – this applies especially to teenagers
- Medic alert bracelets, steroid cards, warfarin books.

Cardinal sins of communication

- NOT LISTENING.
- Asking questions too soon in the consultation.
- Rushing the patient.
- Looking bored and showing disinterest.
- Being patronising, dictatorial or rude.
- Making assumptions that are incorrect and unsupported by the information gained.
- Ignoring cultural sensitivities.

 Tip – Always write down the specifics of the patient information given. Just writing *leaflet given* or *risks discussed* is not sufficient.

LEGAL GUIDANCE – INFORMED CONSENT AND ADULTS WITH CAPACITY

This section deals with adult patients (those of 18 years or over) and those who are not detained under the Mental Health Act. Detained patients and children will be dealt with later.

There are two categories of patient in the informed consent arena:

- those who have the mental capacity to make a decision
- those who lack the mental capacity to make a decision.

The way in which doctors may treat patients depends on the category into which the patient falls.

Patients who have capacity

Patients who have capacity have autonomy; they may make any decision they want to. They can even refuse life-saving treatment.

If a doctor treats a patient who has capacity against their wishes, or without first obtaining proper informed consent, he can be disciplined by his employer, charged with a criminal offence, sued through the civil courts and struck off the medical register.

Patients who lack capacity

These patients are treated under the doctrine of emergency or the principle of **best interests**. The Mental Capacity Act 2005 (in Scotland: the Adults with Incapacity (Scotland) Act 2000) gives more detail on how the law works with patients who lack capacity (for example, if the patient has appointed a lasting power of attorney). This will be discussed in detail later in the section *Informed consent and adults who lack capacity*.

How do I assess capacity?

The Mental Capacity Act sets out the test for capacity. It is a two-stage process.

Stage 1 of assessing capacity

In order to declare a patient incapacitous, you must first judge them to be suffering from: **an impairment of, or disturbance in, the mind or brain**.

Decide whether it is the mind or the brain that you consider to be impaired. For example, would you say that a patient with a diagnosis of bipolar disorder, who is in a manic phase, is suffering an impairment of, or a disturbance in their mind **or** their brain? What about someone who has had a severe stroke?

 Tip – You do not need to do a formal capacity assessment on every patient. You only have to do an assessment if there is something to suggest you should, e.g. the patient has a diagnosis of a mental illness or is crying uncontrollably. This is because there is a presumption of capacity in UK law.

If you believe a patient to be suffering from an impairment of, or disturbance in, the mind or brain, you can move onto the second stage. Otherwise, you must decide that a patient **has** capacity.

Stage 2 of assessing capacity

Ask yourself whether the patient can:
- retain the treatment information
- understand it

- use or weigh up the information as part of the process of making a decision
- communicate their decision.

A person may be declared incapacitous if he fails only one of the above criteria. If you decide a patient lacks capacity you must record how you came to your decision with reference to the two-stage test.

 Tip – If a patient has fluctuating capacity, for example someone with a diagnosis of Alzheimer's, who has lucid or good days, consider obtaining an advanced statement from them on one of their good days. Advanced statements will be discussed in the *Informed consent and adults who lack capacity* section, p. 16.

 Tip – Always ask patients to repeat back the treatment information. Never ask patients if they have understood you. Most will say yes, even if they didn't.

Always ask patients why they want to go ahead with a proposed treatment and record their rationale in the records. This will make it easier to manage a patient's expectations.

 Tip – If you are not sure whether a patient has capacity:
- ask a colleague for their view
- contact the Mental Health Liaison Team
- call your in-house legal department.

If you are unsure of capacity, you should only proceed with treatment in an emergency. Emergency situations are discussed in: *Informed consent and adults who lack capacity*, p. 16.

Capacity is **decision specific**. This means that patients may have capacity to consent to some treatments or interventions, but not to others. The more serious the implications, the higher the level of capacity required.

For example – a patient with moderate learning disabilities may lack capacity to consent for surgery to remove their appendix, but have capacity to consent to their blood pressure being taken.

Treatment of patients who have capacity

Patients with capacity can make any decision they want to. Before they do so you must make sure that any decision they make is **voluntary and informed**.

Voluntary decisions by patients

You must be satisfied that treatment decisions are taken without coercion. This includes coercion by the health professional, friends and family members. If, for example, you think that a patient's family is putting pressure on them to receive a certain treatment, it is a good idea to try to speak to the patient without their family present and to find out their personal wishes.

If you are faced with an elderly patient who is happy to go along with anything you suggest, you may wish to spend some time satisfying yourself that they are making a decision based on their own feelings rather than on the basis of trying to please you or not wanting to cause a fuss.

Informed decisions by patients

You must tell patients about:
- significant risks and possible side effects
- benefits

- alternative treatments
- any aspect of the treatment to which the patient, because of his or her personality or circumstances, would be likely to attach significance – this is called **material information**.

An example of material information would be if a patient should not get their scar wet for a number of weeks after their operation. This may be of particular importance to someone who is a competitive swimmer.

The amount and type of information required by a patient will be different in every case, and even very small risks (less than 1% chance of something happening) may be of importance to a particular patient.

 Tip – It is good practice to take a detailed history from a patient and find out what their personal circumstances are. Ask what they do for a living and ask yourself whether you need to emphasise any bits of information.
A note of information discussed with a patient might read – *Went through information leaflet 22 with Mr Brown. In particular, I emphasised that he would not be able to drive for 3 months. He is a taxi driver. He said he was prepared to accept this as he is 'fed up with the pain'.*

Do I need to get a patient to sign a consent form?

The validity of consent does not depend on a signed form. Written consent is only evidence of consent: if a decision isn't taken voluntarily, with appropriate information and from someone with capacity, a signature on a form will not make the consent valid.

Although completion of a consent form is in most cases not a legal requirement (exceptions include certain requirements of the Mental Health Act 1983 and of the Human

Fertilisation and Embryology Act 1990), the use of such forms is good practice and is expected by national guidance where an intervention such as surgery is to be undertaken.

If the patient has capacity, and wishes to give consent, but is physically unable to mark the form, this fact should be recorded in the notes. If consent has been validly given, the lack of a completed form is no bar to treatment.

 Tip – You should obtain written consent when a patient participates in a research project or a video recording (even if only minor procedures are involved).

LEGAL GUIDANCE – INFORMED CONSENT AND ADULTS WHO LACK CAPACITY

The Mental Capacity Act 2005, which came into force in 2007, governs the treatment of adults in England and Wales who lack capacity to make their own choices. This Act sets out the legal test for capacity (see *Informed consent and adults with capacity*, p. 11, for guidance on capacity assessment). In Scotland the Adults with Incapacity (Scotland) Act 2000 applies.

Emergency treatment

Patients may be treated in emergency situations where it is not possible for them to give consent (perhaps because they are unconscious or in considerable pain).

The legal principle is that patients may be treated in a defined emergency to prevent a serious deterioration in either their physical or mental health, but that there should be no treatment under this principle that goes beyond the point of crisis.

Any treatment that falls outside this definition must be administered under the doctrine of **best interests**, which will be discussed later in this section, p. 18.

The important point to note here is that doctors must be sure to document what constituted the emergency and what serious deterioration they were seeking to prevent by treating the patient. They must also make it quite clear that all actions were proportionate. Proportionality can be explained as follows: you must not take a sledge hammer to crack a nut.

Ideally, the patient should make their own decisions. Treating a patient without first talking through how they would wish to be treated, is an infringement of their rights. Thus, if treatment is not urgent and can safely be delayed until the patient regains capacity to make their own choices, then that is precisely what should happen.

You are entitled to use reasonable force to treat under the doctrine of emergency. For example, you can hold down a distressed road traffic victim in order to administer pain killers or apply monitors.

You must always have capacity at the forefront of your mind.

 Tip – You have a positive duty to treat patients who lack the ability to make their own choices.

Case study

Consider a patient who is brought into Accident and Emergency by some friends. He appears to have been drinking heavily. He is also bleeding profusely from a cut to his hand. A superficial review tells you he appears to have severed some tendons and without immediate intervention will suffer long-term injury. He keeps brushing you off and clearly wants to leave the unit. He is not being violent, but clearly is reluctant to be touched.

It is probable that his capacity to make a decision about his treatment has been affected by the alcohol he has drunk. The fact that his incapacity is self-inflicted is irrelevant. You may therefore use reasonable force to treat him. But be sure to document the force used and the necessity for it carefully in the notes. Force should only be used as a last resort.

> You should NEVER use physical force to treat someone with capacity (note the exception of the detained patient, p. 81).

Non-urgent treatment and best interests

The principle which applies in non-urgent situations is the doctrine of **best interests**. This doctrine, which is now set out in the Mental Capacity Act 2005, enables you to treat a patient who lacks capacity, as long as the treatment is in their best interests.

The doctrine of best interests has **three stages**. First, you must identify all the medical options. There will always be at least two options: do something or do nothing. In most cases there will be more than two options.

The second stage is to list and assess the patient's best interests. An assessment of best interests should not be limited to medical considerations but should include an assessment of the patient's values and preferences expressed when competent (including any advance decision or statement they may have made), their psychological health, well-being, quality of life, and spiritual and religious welfare. Financial interests may also be relevant. You should consult interested parties, any attorney the patient may have appointed, or relatives and friends of the patient, where practicable and appropriate to do so, to help to form a view on best interests. For serious interventions where the patient has no family or friends, you should involve the Independent Mental Capacity Advocate (IMCA) service, (see p. 21 for more details).

You will normally aim to preserve life but this will not always be in a patient's best interests, especially if the patient's general health is very poor and the prognosis is pessimistic. This is because active intervention may mean the burden of treatment outweighs any benefit and could be said to be futile.

The third stage is to choose the most appropriate option and to document your reasoning.

 Tip – If you decide that it is not practicable or appropriate to consult interested parties, you should document your reasons in the notes.

Advance decisions to refuse treatment

An advance decision to refuse treatment:

- can only be made by an adult (18 years old or above) who has the capacity to do so
- must have been made voluntarily, and the patient fully informed of the implications of, and alternatives to, the decision
- should specify a situation where the patient will lack capacity to make a decision, for example, if they lose consciousness
- must specify a treatment modality and expressly state that treatment is not to be started or continued, i.e. must constitute a refusal
- may be withdrawn or altered at any time when a patient has the capacity to do so (a withdrawal does not need to be in writing).

For more information on the validity and applicability of advance decisions, see Section 24 onwards of the Mental Capacity Act 2005.

Advance decisions that are expressed in the positive or otherwise do not meet the requirements of a valid advance decision are known as advance statements. These are persuasive when you are considering what may be in a patient's best interests.

Life-sustaining treatment

An advance decision is not applicable to life-sustaining treatment unless:

- the decision is verified by a statement by the patient to the effect that it is to apply to that treatment even if their life is at risk
- the decision is in writing
- the decision is signed by the patient, or by another person in the patient's presence and at the patient's direction
- the signature is made or acknowledged by the patient in the presence of a witness
- the witness signs it, or acknowledges his signature, in the patient's presence.

Lasting Powers of Attorney

The Mental Capacity Act 2005 creates a new Lasting Power of Attorney which can be used to assign another person the right to make decisions on a patient's behalf relating to:

- health
- welfare
- property
- money.

The Attorney must always act in a donee's, i.e. the patient's, best interests. This is the same test as that which would be applied to a clinician's decision.

The format of a Lasting Power of Attorney is set out in Schedule 1, Part 1, of the Mental Capacity Act 2005. Although broadly similar, the law in Scotland is slightly different and is found in the Adults with Incapacity (Scotland) Act 2000.

Deputies

If a doctor is faced with family members who all have different and strong views they will have to consider obtaining a single order from the Court of Protection (England and Wales only) to resolve the dispute or, in rarer cases, the appointment of a deputy. A Deputy is a court-appointed advocate.

If a patient has not appointed someone to make healthcare decisions on their behalf by way of a Lasting Power of Attorney, the Court of Protection may appoint a Deputy. However, the Deputy's appointment is likely to be very limited in scope and duration.

Deputies are likely to be appointed in rare cases, for example, '... *where there is a dispute between family members as to who has the patient's best interests at heart and where the patient has chronic and/ or degenerative health problems calling for repeated assessments and decisions by doctors and carers...*' (Government response to recommendation 54 of the Joint Committee's report).

It is likely that the Deputy will have some relationship to the patient. If there is a Lasting Power of Attorney any disputes must be resolved by way of a Single Order of the Court rather than the appointment of a Deputy.

Independent Advocates

The Mental Capacity Act set up a new service called the Independent Mental Capacity Advocate (IMCA). IMCAs help people who have no family or friends. A doctor will have a duty to contact an IMCA if there is no one they can talk to about the person's best interests.

Court of Protection (England and Wales only)

The new Court of Protection created by the Mental Capacity Act has a comprehensive jurisdiction over the health, welfare and financial affairs of people who lack capacity.

The Court of Protection may make orders of the following kind:

- Declarations as to capacity
- Declarations as to best interests (Single Orders)
- Appointment of a deputy
- Declarations as to the validity of Lasting Powers of Attorney
- Orders relating to financial matters (Single Orders)
- Declaration as to the lawfulness or otherwise of any act done, or yet to be done, in relation to a patient
- Declaration as to the existence, validity and applicability of advance decisions.

Office of the Public Guardian

The Public Guardian helps the Court of Protection by looking after the applications and paperwork for Lasting Powers of Attorney and Deputies. Additionally, the Public Guardian will monitor the work of Deputies, and works with the Police and Social Services if it is suspected that a vulnerable person is being abused.

Court of Protection Visitors

The Lord Chancellor may appoint Special Visitors (clinicians) and general visitors (who are not clinicians). The role of visitors will be to visit and carry out independent reports on matters relating to the exercising of powers under the Mental Capacity Act. They have the power to see and take copies of medical records and to see the patient in private.

Scottish Position

 Although broadly similar to the approach adopted in England and Wales, there are a few differences of note in Scotland. The law in this area is governed by the Adults with Incapacity (Scotland) Act 2000. Unlike in England and Wales, the principle of **best interests** is not the central theme for treating patients without capacity. Instead there are a number of **factors** that must be taken into account. The 2000 Act grants a practitioner with primary responsibility for a patient a **general authority to treat** a person who, in the practitioner's opinion, is incapable of taking a decision. A proxy can be appointed under the 2000 Act, but while they can consent to treatment, they have no power to refuse treatment on behalf of the patient.

Further reading

- Department of Health – Good practice in consent implementation guide: consent to examination or treatment*
- Department of Health – Reference guide to consent for examination or treatment*
- Department of Health – Model policy for consent to examination or treatment*
- British Medical Association – Consent tool kit, 2nd edition
- Code of Practice for the Mental Capacity Act.

  * *Note:* This document has not been updated since the introduction of the MCA.

BREAKING BAD NEWS

Breaking bad news is a very particular form of communication and an essential skill for the practice of medicine. It is often tested in clinical finals, and at least one practical OSCE station will generally be based on this core skill. Getting it right is therefore crucial. Below are helpful tips for delivering news that has potentially life-changing consequences for the patient and their family.

Setting the scene

- **Where** – a quiet room away from the busy ward so that privacy is possible. Provide comforts in the room: cups of tea/coffee, tissues and good seating.
- **When –** a dedicated slot of time when you're not likely to be disturbed.
- **Who –** decide who should be present, e.g. advocacy services/ nurses/ yourself/senior person. It is a good idea to bring in a member of the team or nursing staff, so they can act as a witness and document contemporaneous notes while the news is given. The named nurse may be able to act as a support for the patient, as someone who has provided care earlier.
- **How** – remove your bleep/switch off your mobile phone and tell the ward staff that you'll be breaking bad news, where you are and not to disturb you.
- **What –** carry information packs, relevant to the condition, in your pocket.
- Ask the patient if they would like someone to accompany them.

The delivery of bad news

- Check the patient's or family's understanding first and what information they are expecting and/or have been told previously. This provides a solid base for delivery of information.

- Ask them if they would like to know more and give a warning about the nature of the news *(this is bad news...*or *I have some difficult information to tell you....).*
- Acknowledge the severity of the situation as appropriate.
- If they want to know more, have the facts clear in your own mind and mentally present the information to yourself first.
- Deliver the information at the **personal** pace of the patient and allow for pauses.
- Use unambiguous words, avoid *erm* or *er*, to sound more professional.
- Wait for the response. This may be highly variable, ranging from crying to taking it on the chin but, whatever the response, give the patient time to gather their thoughts.
- You can talk about a disease **if they want.** However, the emphasis should initially be on the **positive aspects**, e.g. HIV: *most people can expect to lead a normal life and, with the development of increasingly effective drugs, life expectancy is getting nearer that of the average person.*
- There is a fine balance between misleading the patient by being too positive, and honesty, even if that honesty is brutal.

Above all, be honest, open, frank and receptive to the patient's speech and body language.

After breaking the bad news

- If the patient clearly cannot tolerate more information, then it is best to end the consultation and allow time for information consolidation. Say: *Clearly this is a lot to take in – let me give you some time to digest the news.*

- Ask if they have further questions and be honest if you don't know the answer, especially regarding prognosis. Tell the patient that you will endeavour to find out the answers, or find someone who can address those issues.
- Reassure the patient by saying what will happen in the future, e.g. making their life as comfortable as possible, referring them to another team or awaiting more tests.
- Offer counselling services, e.g. bereavement services.
- Offer any leaflets/handouts that may be useful.
- Ask if any religious support could be useful.
- Offer them your contact number for further questions and make sure you return the call!
- Offer details of lay support groups (local or national).

2 Communication-specific scenarios

LEGAL GUIDANCE – PATIENT CONFIDENTIALITY

Overview: Respecting a patient's wishes

The general rule is that patient information, including pictures, photographs or other images, should not be disclosed in a form that might identify the patient, unless they have given informed consent.

There are some exceptions to this rule (see p. 30) but your starting point should always be to respect patient confidentiality. This means that you should always tell a patient what you intend to do with their information.

Example

Before sending a discharge letter to a GP, get the patient's consent. If the patient objects, then you should respect their decision. You should, however, take the time to explain the implications of the decision, namely that their care may be compromised or even withdrawn.

Practical points

- You should not take patient records home.
- Always log out of a computer when you are finished.
- Clear your screen of one patient's information before seeing another.
- Do not share your login or password.

 Tip – Get into the habit of discussing confidentiality with every new patient.
You do not need to obtain informed consent for every disclosure necessary to provide care, provided a patient understands:
- what information will be held about them
- how it will be held

- who will have access to it
- that they have the choice to limit how the information is used or shared and consent.

If a patient lacks mental capacity (p. 16) to make choices about the use of their information, you may share their information if this is necessary to provide care and it is in the patient's best interests.

You must get explicit informed consent and a signature from the patient if you intend to use patient-identifiable information for research or teaching.

 Tip – Use the NHS leaflet on patient confidentiality and information disclosure to inform your discussions. Ask whether the patient has any questions. If they do and you do not know the answer, refer them to someone who can help.

Exceptions

There are times when you are able to disclose patient information without consent or against the express wishes of a patient.

The following is an overview of a very complex area of law. If you are contemplating a disclosure for anything other than treatment or care purposes and you do not have consent, you should obtain legal advice. You can get this from your Defence Union or your organisation's legal department.

The following govern the law on confidentiality:

- Data Protection Act 1998 (DPA)
- Human Rights Act 1998 (HRA)
- Common law

- Professional guidance
- Caldicott principles
- Public Health (Infectious Diseases) Regulations 1988 (PHIDR)
- Access to Health Records Act 1990 (AHRA) which governs access to health records of deceased patients.

What is common law?

 Common law is the set of legal principles that build up on a subject as a result of individual cases being brought. This is distinct from Statute, where an Act of Parliament (such as the Mental Capacity Act) sets out the legal principles on a subject. Often common law and Statutes will stand alongside each other, with individual cases being brought on points of statute interpretation. For example, the case of Diane Pretty was a high-profile challenge against the law that anyone convicted of helping someone take his or her own life faces a jail term of up to 14 years. Mrs Pretty, who had motor neurone disease, wanted an assurance that her husband would not be prosecuted if he helped her to take her own life. Her challenge was unsuccessful.

Case studies and examples

Case Study 1 – Disclosure of a deceased patient's records

If someone asks to see the medical records of a deceased patient you must first check that they are entitled to make the request. The AHRA states that only a personal representative, executor of the deceased's estate or someone who has a claim arising out of the death may apply for access. You will need to see a copy of the grant of probate or letters of administration before releasing the records.

Case Study 2 – Disclosure to the police

It will rarely be the case that you will have good reason to disclose patient information to the police without a court order or patient consent.

If a police officer asks to see a patient's records you should ask them to set out the reason for their request in writing. Explain that you do not wish to be obstructive but that you want to seek legal advice.

Case Study 3 – Disclosure to protect others

If you believe that a failure to release certain information would expose another individual to risk of death or serious harm you may disclose to the appropriate authorities.

- You would normally tell the patient of your intention to disclose unless to do so would prejudice the purpose.
- You may also be justified in disclosing information to prevent or detect a crime.
- You should obtain legal advice before undertaking such a disclosure.

You may notify the DVLA if you believe a patient's continued car usage is putting others at risk. You should tell the patient of your intention before disclosing. You should only disclose the minimum information necessary.

Case Study 4 – Disclosure of a child's information to parents

If a child asks you not to tell their parents that they have sought and received treatment you should try to respect their wishes. However, you may disregard the child's request if you think that maintaining confidentiality would not be in the child's best interests.

You should tell the child of your intention and if necessary put them in contact with a Patient Advice and Liaison Services (PALS) representative.

PALS provide information, advice and support to help patients, families and their carers. Every trust should have a PALS representative.

Further reading

- NHS Code of Practice – Confidentiality
- GMC Guidance on Confidentiality
- Working Together to Safeguard Children.

EXPLAINING RESULTS

All doctors will have to explain test results to patients or their relatives, so it is necessary to have a good idea how to do so well. Doctors must also use their judgement in deciding if the news they will give is good or bad. The reaction of the patient will depend upon the rapport they have developed previously with their clinician.

There are essentially two types of result: those which have definitive consequences and those where no answer can be given at the moment.

Discussing definitive test results

In situations where the results of blood tests, X-rays, scans etc. provide a diagnosis:

- Introduce yourself to the patient.
- Refresh the patient's memory of the tests that they've had so far.
- Find out the patient's prior knowledge of the tests they've had and explore their expectations.
- Tell them what the results are in an unambiguous way and explain their immediate implications.

- Explain the disease and the management plan, including:
  - which specialists the patient needs to see
  - how long the plan would take and length of stay in hospital
  - any more tests that need to be done
  - any medication that needs to be started.

For example, you could say – *Your heart scan has shown that your heart failure has worsened since your last scan 3 years ago. What the team suggests is to modify your tablets and increase the dose of furosemide. We hope this will get rid of the excess fluid. We would like you to come back in 2 months' time for an outpatient check up with Dr X.*

When tests do not lead to a definitive answer

This is a highly awkward scenario because, understandably, the patient will be anxious about their health, believe that they are actively suffering with a symptom or from a condition, and want to know the cause.

In situations where the results of tests do not provide a diagnosis:

- Understand the patient's angle; lack of closure and imperfect answers are most distressing.
- Start off by refreshing the patient's memory of the tests they had.
- Say that the tests have not shown anything conclusive and it is therefore difficult to deduce anything meaningful from them, but that this does not mean the doctors are going to give up.
- Suggest further courses of action, which could be:
  - to review all the blood tests and results so far to see if anything has been missed
  - to refer to particular specialists or to a colleague for a second opinion

- the use of multidisciplinary meetings where all types of specialist can be present and give an opinion
- to carry out further, more complicated or specific tests, e.g. scans/blood tests, etc.

> If a patient has capacity (p. 11) you must first obtain their consent before discussing results and prognosis with relatives.

COMMUNICATING WITH CHILDREN

Younger child

Trying to take a detailed history from young children can be very hard, since the majority are shy of strangers and they may have short attention spans. If they show understanding, try to involve them in their care.

- Throughout taking a history from the parent/carer/ guardian, try to confirm the story with the child and gauge their reaction.
- Distract the child with toys if need be. This can be very useful in assessing the child's neurological status and their developmental level in relation to their chronological age. It will also allow you to engage the parent and discuss any concerns the parents may have, without them being distracted by their child.
- Always explain to the child what is going to happen to them (but in basic language) and use comparisons to everyday events, e.g. photo/picture of their tummy for abdominal X-ray.

Parents of young children can be incredibly concerned about their child's health, so take on board their concerns. Remember the old adage that a mother knows her child best. If their concerns are unwarranted, reassuring the parents will go a long way to developing a good relationship between you and the family. It may even calm the child, if they can see that their parent or guardian is calmer and more relaxed.

Use picture diagrams or even dolls as ways of communication. These can be used to assess severity of pain, anatomical location of complaints, etc.

Older child

Children, especially those nearing adolescence, will behave more like an adult. They can concentrate more and are able to explain more, with a wider vocabulary. They may be treated in a more adult way than a younger child. Some 11–12 year olds may be treated like adolescents (see *Communicating with young people (adolescents)* below), but parental involvement is still very important and should always be actively encouraged.

- Children of this age are at school. Always ask the parent/guardian about their progress at school, how well they make friends, if they are bullied or have been suspended/expelled.
- Clarify with the child. They may be shy about this, but a little gentle persistence generally pays off. Difficulties at school may present as physical symptoms and/or exacerbate current medical problems.
- Again, as in the younger age group, explaining things in simple terms using everyday comparisons may prove useful.

Communicating with young people (adolescents)

This group is perceived to be difficult because:
- they can be unsure of self-identity and are still developing their own thoughts and health beliefs
- there may be pressure to conform to their peers and so appear not to be different

- lack of foresight and maturity may lead to a lack of understanding of the effects of chronic disease in later years, e.g. diabetes mellitus.

With adolescents try:

- being flexible
- allowing teenagers to voice suggestions about management and getting them to cooperate
- not to patronise
- not to be dictatorial/autocratic (e.g. *You **must** take your insulin twice a day on time...*)
- not to talk to parents directly/exclusively when agreeing an adolescent's management and therefore ignoring the adolescent patient's concerns
- accepting adolescents' autonomy
- allowing peers/friends to join the consultation, not always insisting on an adult companion
- showing empathy about how the patient might be viewed by their peers and family
- focusing on how the adolescent can accommodate any management into their very individual lifestyles.

Legal Guidance – Treating children for physical conditions*

Whilst adults with mental capacity to do so can make any treatment decision they want, the situation is somewhat different with children. For treatment purposes, a child is defined as anyone under the age of 18 (see Guidance box: Scottish law, below).

A person with parental responsibility can give consent (i.e. say *yes*) to treatment (and indeed to an examination) but they do not have the absolute right to refuse treatment or examination, i.e. to say *no*.

---

* *Note*: For treatment of children for mental disorder, see MHA Code of Practice, Part 36.

Parental responsibility

Parental responsibility is conferred automatically on the mother of a child, irrespective of her marital status. Whether the father also has parental responsibility depends on whether he was married to the mother at the time of the child's birth. If he was married to the mother, then he will also have automatic parental responsibility. If the couple were not married, the father may acquire parental responsibility in one of the following ways:

- making a parental responsibility agreement with the mother
- obtaining a parental responsibility order from the court
- obtaining a residence order from the court
- being appointed the child's guardian by the court, by the mother or by another guardian
- for children born after 1 December 2003 – by registering the child's birth jointly with the mother at the time of birth.

You do not need to conduct a formal mental capacity assessment (p. 12) on the person with parental responsibility before taking their consent, unless there is something to suggest that you should – for example, if they are very tearful or otherwise appear distressed. This is because adults are presumed in law to have capacity.

Reminder of capacity assessments

You must ask yourself whether the individual can:

- retain the treatment information
- understand it
- use or weigh the information as part of the process of making a decision
- communicate their decision.

Both 16- and 17-year-old children can say *yes* but do not have the right to give you a binding *no*. They are also presumed in law to have capacity. This means that you do not have to undertake a formal capacity assessment on them unless there is something to suggest that you should.

This contrasts with children under the age of 16. These younger children can still give you a valid *yes* (although not an absolute *no*) but you must undertake and document a formal capacity assessment on them before relying on their consent alone. There is no presumption of capacity for children under 16, who, if found to have capacity, are described as being **Gillick competent**.

Gillick competence

The phrase 'Gillick competence' derives from a case of that name in which a GP prescribed the contraceptive pill to a 15-year-old without consulting her parents. His actions were deemed lawful since he had respected the welfare principle and the child had mental capacity to make her own choices. Sometimes a Gillick competent child is referred to as a **Fraser guideline child** after the Judge in the Gillick case. It means the same thing. *Gillick v West Norfolk and Wisbech Area Health Authority* [1985] 3 All ER 402 (HL).

The reason why there is a difference between a *yes* and a *no* with children, but not with adults, is because of the **welfare principle**. This legal concept states that the welfare of the child must come first. This principle overrides all other principles, including the principle of autonomy.

Scottish law – legal capacity

The age of legal capacity in Scotland is 16 years. Consent by children in Scotland is governed by the Age of Legal Capacity (Scotland) Act 1991. A child under 16 can consent to their own medical treatment where, *in the opinion of a qualified medical practitioner, they are capable of understanding the nature and possible consequences of the procedure or treatment.* This places Gillick competence on a statutory footing. It has not been authoritatively determined by the Scottish Courts whether a child under 16 has a right to **refuse** consent. In the absence of such authority, English law must be seen as persuasive, which would suggest a parent could still consent.

Different views

Theoretically, in England and Wales, in law you only need one consent. So, if a competent child is saying *yes* but a parent is saying *no* (or vice versa) you could rely on the single *yes*. This has not been authoritatively established in Scotland. However, in practice you should proceed with extreme caution and should certainly obtain advice. This is because a disagreement may suggest that you have not properly assessed what is in the child's best interests. The principle of best interests is not limited to medical necessity but extends to all aspects of life. In serious cases, a declaration should be sought from the Courts as to what is in a child's best interests.

 Tip – When documenting a 'best interests' assessment consider organising your notes as follows:
- List all the medical options.
- List the best interest considerations such as school work, hobbies, etc.
- State which option is most appropriate, bearing in mind the clinical standpoint and the wider best-interests context.

Child attending alone

It is lawful to treat a child in the absence of their parents. This is because a child with capacity can give consent on his or her own behalf. Alternatively, you may think that delaying treatment of a child who lacks capacity, until the parents can be contacted, would not be in the best interests of the child. In most cases you should, however, request a chaperone.

Telling the parents

There will be times when a child does not want their parents to know about their treatment. Such a request constitutes a refusal, a *no*, and as such you do not have to respect it. That said, you must weigh up whether telling the parents really is in the child's best interests. Is there another relative you could inform? What about a teacher? You should always seek the advice of a colleague before breaching confidentiality against a competent child's wishes. You should also tell the child your intentions.

The rights of the fetus

An unborn child does not have rights; only when it is born alive does it acquire them. Once born alive, it has rights in relation to any harm caused to it whilst in the womb. Where the unborn child is not successfully born, there can be no action arising from any acts harming the fetus, as it never became a legal person. Additionally, the father of a fetus has no rights in respect of its care. It is for the mother alone to decide how she wants to be treated.

COMMUNICATING WITH OTHER SPECIAL PATIENT GROUPS

Communicating with elderly patients

Elderly patients may often have multiple problems, which can make communication difficult. Particular impairments may include:
- dementia: poor memory retention and understanding
- depression
- multiple medical problems
- poor sight
- poor hearing
- poor mobility.

When communicating with elderly patients try:

- consistent and constant education to reinforce any advice and not confuse the patient. This is particularly important for chronic diseases, such as cardiovascular disease, where the regime can include three or four different drugs

- talking slowly and slightly louder than normal, and enunciating each word clearly for those who are hard of hearing (but beware of being seen to be treating a patient as simple)
- using diagrams and written information to take away
- suggesting that the patient bring a companion or family member who can act as an advocate, or even be involved in the management with the patient's consent
- allowing more time for the consultation
- not dismissing what they have to say as elderly idle chatter.

Hearing impaired patients

Remember that being deaf does not always mean complete hearing loss. When communicating with hearing impaired patients try:

- having a light source on your face, so the patient can see your mouth clearly. Most deaf people can lip read well
- exaggerating your facial movements when speaking and speaking more slowly than normal (do not speak excessively loudly: it can appear that you are shouting)
- reducing background noise in the room, especially for those with hearing aids
- having someone accompany the patient, with their consent, to act as a 'second pair of ears'
- learning basic sign language
- writing down key words so the patient has a visual prompt
- giving out leaflets
- advising of the availability of a loop system.

Visually impaired patients

Remember that being registered blind does not necessarily imply a complete loss of vision.

When communicating with visually impaired patients, remember that it is imperative to remain within the patient's visual field and try:

- asking politely if they can see you or any written words and adjust your behaviour accordingly
- asking whether they need your help (offer rather than assume)
- guiding them to a chair and, if appropriate, using touch to attract their attention
- allowing guide dogs to be present in consultations
- avoiding classic faux pas, for example saying: *as you can see…*
- using Braille leaflets and Braille door signs
- organising an appropriate interpreter for deaf–blind patients.

Patients whose first language is not English

- If the practice area is known to have a high ethnic population, learn a few basic phrases.
- Have a translation sheet for common ailments and common conditions (you obviously need to check that the patient has a basic level of literacy).
- Use advocates and translators approved by the Health Trust. It can take time to secure services, so plan ahead. There are translator telephones available which can be used as a translation service.
- You should only use family members as translators in exceptional circumstances where the delay in finding an official translator is likely to cause harm and where the patient agrees. We strongly advise against using children as translators, particularly for intimate examinations or where there is any suggestion whatsoever that the patient may wish to discuss intimate matters with you. For example, a woman may wish to talk about a

gynaecological problem but not want to discuss it in front of her child.

Physically disabled patients

- Ask if they want their carer to accompany them during the consultation.
- Converse with the patient directly and not the carer.
- Have the desk at an appropriate height for wheelchairs and wide enough spaces around the desk and room to allow easy access.
- Respect the patient's dignity and allow extra time for undressing/dressing themselves for examinations and moving to the examination couch. Remember the limits these patients may have in their bodily movements – having a classic examination position may be not practical.

Ethnic and cultural diversity

- Women may express a preference to be seen by a female doctor, especially when wanting to discuss female health issues.
- Muslim patients prefer same-gender consultations and in some quarters regard the Western greeting formality as too forward.
- Jewish patients – some of the more Orthodox Jewish sects need female GPs for women patients.

EXPLAINING PATIENT DISCHARGE (FOUNDATION YEAR LEVEL)

It is a primary duty of house officers to facilitate a smooth discharge, following a hospital admission.

Background work

Write the discharge letters and prescriptions early so that patients aren't waiting for a long time (or even until the next day) for the medication to be delivered from the pharmacy.

Before the date of discharge, liaise with the nursing staff and other health professionals regarding any potential discharge problems, e.g. social or rehabilitation issues that may need to be addressed.

Speaking to the patient

Introduce yourself and remind the patient of the earlier decision to discharge. Ask the patient how they feel about being discharged. This is important – patients may not want to go home because of ongoing pain, no one to pick them up, no food in the house, or they may be worried that their house is unheated. Explore the reasons why they may be apprehensive. Most patients are, however, generally keen to go home.

If they agree to discharge, make sure that the following information is covered:

- Explain that the reasons for admission have been resolved or that the patient is stable enough to be discharged home.
- Explain that a discharge letter has been written. They will need to keep one copy for themselves and deliver the other to their GP at a later date.
- Explain any medication they will be going home with, the purpose of the drug and any side effects to watch out for. They can wait for their medication or go home and come back for it later.
- Ask if they need a sick note for time off work, or any other letters to confirm their admission.
- Tell them of any follow-up plans such as:

- GP follow-up, consultant follow-up, or referrals to other departments (appointments are generally sent through the post)
- any scans or procedures they need before appointments
- any other health professional staff who are to be involved in care, e.g. nurse specialists, district nurse, physiotherapist, and what they will be doing and how to contact them.
- Tell them of any social issues that have been addressed before discharge, e.g. meals on wheels in place, daily carer to come in to help wash and clothe, nursing home placement booked, key worker assigned and if other works to be done, e.g. changing parts of the house.
- Inform them of any other issues that need to be addressed in the future.
- Surgical patients on discharge need to be told when clips/sutures will be removed (normally a week/10 days), who will do that (district nurse/GP), how long they need to be off work (normally 1–2 weeks).
- Advise patients to seek certification from their GP for work absence.
- Tell them that if they become worse suddenly they need to come back to A&E as soon as possible or seek advice from their GP. Give examples of what to look out for.
- Give them any information leaflets that they may require, such as head injury advice.

DEALING WITH POTENTIAL SELF-DISCHARGING PATIENTS (FOUNDATION YEAR LEVEL)

Why people self discharge:
- Impatience while waiting for treatment/drugs
- Perceived lack of effectiveness of treatment

- Poor rapport with nursing and medical staff
- Influenced by family and friends
- Intoxication with illicit drugs/alcohol
- Own beliefs regarding treatment and personality issues.

Self-discharge, a typical scenario

Often you will receive a call from another healthcare professional, such as a nurse, stating that a patient is threatening to self-discharge. Tell the nurse to ask the patient to wait until you arrive.

Once you are with the patient:

- Tell the patient that the team believes that the patient should stay for treatment. Explain that it would not be medically safe for them to leave and why. Set out the clinical reasons why they should stay, e.g. need scan, blood test results, another specialist's opinion.
- Apologise for any delay in getting scans done/blood tests reported, etc.
- Repeat what the management plan is again and explore whether there is anything the team can do to improve the situation.
- Negotiate with the patient, e.g. – *If we can't do the scan by tomorrow, I'll talk to my team about alternative arrangements.*
- Inform them politely that once they leave, the hospital and its staff relinquish all legal liability for their health because they're going against the doctors' advice, but be careful when doing so not to come across as threatening or coercive.

The competent adult has the legal right to refuse treatment and leave. If they want to go despite requests to stay, you need to let them go.

- Before they leave, ensure they sign a special self-discharge form with a witness (usually ward sister).
- Document in the notes all matters pertaining to the incident and inform the GP.

Legal Guidance – Self-discharge

Self-discharge is effectively a refusal of treatment. Accordingly, all the principles of informed consent apply. The overriding principle of informed consent is that an adult patient with mental capacity can make any decision they want to – even a decision you think is silly.

When an adult patient indicates a desire to self-discharge the first thing you need to do is assess their mental capacity to make that decision. For guidance on mental capacity decisions in general, see *Treatment of patients who have capacity*, p. 14.

In particular, you must assess the patient's ability to understand the implications of their decision to leave before they are medically discharged. It is good practice to make a verbatim record of the reason given by the patient for their decision.

You must carefully document your discussion about the specific risks associated with the self-discharge and in many NHS Trusts you are required to ask that the patient sign a self-discharge form. Many of these forms do not provide space for doctors to record capacity assessments or risk discussions and so these should be documented in the health record. A self-discharge form is unlikely, on its own, to protect you. If a person refuses to sign a self-discharge form, you should record this fact and any reason given by the patient for their refusal.

The healthcare team should arrange for transport, where required, and provide the patient with medication, dressings and so on. The patient's GP and any other interested profes-sional should be informed.

DEALING WITH ANGRY PATIENTS AND RELATIVES (FOUNDATION YEAR LEVEL)

Why do patients or relatives become angry and aggressive?

Patients and their relatives lose their temper for a wide range of reasons:

- Frustration from lack of effective treatment, e.g. inadequate pain control
- Medical professionals' attitude, including perceived lack of respect
- A perceived medical mistake such as side effects of the drug/surgery/procedure with feelings of regret or misinformation
- A genuine medical mistake, e.g. wrong dose of medication
- Grief or emotional reaction to a test result
- Personal problems such as pressure from family and relatives or financial difficulties. A sudden illness can lead to great stress in patients and those who are close to them
- Perception of not being properly informed or poor communication with the medical team.

How to do deal with angry patients or relatives

- If you know the person you will be talking to is angry, it is perfectly justifiable to bring someone in with you, e.g. a security guard or a nurse. They can also act as witness for any incidents and act as a deterrent.
- Let the person vent their anger by listening to what they have to say and, if you need to, leave them alone to cool off.

- Remain objective, calm and collected. A person may throw personal insults, but very often it is really the situation that makes them angry and not the person they are insulting.
- Don't try reasoning with angry people: it doesn't work and may cause them to become even angrier.
- Be empathic and explore why the patient or relative feels angry – *I can see you're clearly very angry. Is there more to this?*
- Say you are sorry that the patient feels the way they do. This single empathic act can often reduce formal complaints and proceedings against staff and the NHS. However, do not under any circumstances admit liability. Liability is a legal issue and, as such, is a very different issue from expressing understanding of a patient's anger.
- Offer appropriate medical solutions, such as giving them an update of their care, increasing their dose of analgesia, offering to hurry up the process of scan reporting, etc.
- Do not blame your colleagues or other professionals, even if it does seem that someone is at fault. It's not your role to judge.
- If the patient wants to complain, give information about the process and the contact number of the Patient Advisory Liaison Service (PALS).
- Violence, swearing or aggressive and threatening hand movements and body language are unacceptable and should not be tolerated. You are perfectly within your rights to stop any consultation if you feel unsafe. If violence occurs, call security and speak to the police about possible assault/battery charges. Your legal department should help you with this.
- Document incidents and action plan fully in the patient's notes.

DEALING WITH INTROSPECTIVE PATIENTS (FOUNDATION YEAR LEVEL)

Why do patients become introspective?

There are a whole host of reasons for patients being introspective:

- Depression or grief
- Deafness
- Personality and natural shyness; some people are naturally introverted and medical consultations are not going to change them
- Prior experience of stigma regarding their condition, or embarrassment in what they expect the disease to be
- Wanting to hide the truth, e.g. poor compliance with medication
- Fear and anxiety of doctor, the situation or the outcome.

How to interview introspective patients:

- If fear and anxiety are obvious, try to put the patient at ease by giving good news first.
- Give the patient time to explain themselves and be even more attentive than usual.
- If necessary become their shoulder to cry on.
- Repeat questions throughout the interview, this may help glean more information.
- Explain the consequences of withholding information – *I can only make a very rough guess at your medical problem* or *My not having all the facts could delay a full diagnosis.*
- Suggest reasons why they're introspective – *Are you depressed? Has something bad happened in your life recently? Are the other kids bullying you at school?* and treat depression, if likely.
- Give them a way forward – *I would like you to answer the following questions as fully as you can, but if you're*

uncomfortable with any of them, let me know and we'll move on.

- Offer counselling services if appropriate, e.g. bereavement, domestic violence, or alcohol counselling.
- See section *Hearing impaired patients* p. 42.

DEALING WITH POOR ADHERENCE

Poor adherence is often the number one reason why treatments fail, and the issue needs to be explored before treatment changes are made or management plans amended. The treatment may be the most clinically appropriate but lack efficacy because of poor compliance.

Reasons for poor adherence

- Patients' health beliefs regarding their condition and medication: these can be influenced by friends/family/background reading.
- Patients do not understand the implications of not taking their medication.
- Patients' personality.
- Intolerable side effects.
- Patients are unable to obtain the medication from the chemist due to lack of funds, poor mobility.
- Difficult drug regimes: unable to remember when to take drug, how many pills for each drug, doesn't understand length of course.
- Unable to use a device to administer drug.
- Perceived lack of effectiveness of the drug – *I didn't feel any different so I stopped it.*
- Once symptom free, the patient stops taking the drug because they believe the medication has done its job (e.g. of a course of antibiotics – *Oh, I stopped them after 4 days. I felt a lot better thanks*).

- Poor self image, stigma attached to taking this drug or perception that taking the drug is an admission of fault or personal failure.

How to improve adherence

- Find out why there is poor adherence: do they have difficulty remembering their medications/difficulty in obtaining the medicines etc.?
- Education about:
  - disease (see *Explaining disease X*, p. 107)
  - drugs (see *Explaining drug Y*, p. 145)
  - devices (see *Explaining device Z*, p. 171).
- Social support: e.g. arrangements with pharmacists to deliver drugs to the patients; relative or friend picking up prescriptions; applying for prescription charge exemption; repeat dispensing of prescriptions without a doctor's signature; use of dosset boxes by those with disability; use of Fast Response Teams in hospital.
- Exploring and addressing issues regarding self image, stigma experienced, etc.
- Getting patients to cooperate with management plans through negotiation.
- Information leaflets and other stimuli to jog memory.
- District nurse to come and visit patients to check on adherence.
- Avoiding polypharmacy, particularly in the elderly: use combination drugs to address two medical problems.

3 History taking

GENERAL HISTORY TAKING

Taking the history of a patient is the most important tool you will use in diagnosing a medical problem. To be able to obtain a history that is targeted to the presenting complaint takes practice, as well as knowledge of possible differential diagnoses. In this chapter, we will provide you with a basic structure for asking questions. In the following chapters, we will provide **target questions** to help make a rough diagnosis. These target questions should only be used as a guide, and you should tailor them to your own style. It is also important that the 'physician-driven history-taking approach' must not overwhelm or ignore the patient's agenda and their needs.

General structure

Presenting complaint (PC)

Ask — *What is the main problem that has caused you to come to hospital today?*
　　Find out the main problem/problems that have made this patient present to you. It can sometimes be difficult to pin down the exact symptom(s) making the patient present. If the patient has not come to you directly, find out why they presented to someone else first.

History of the presenting complaint (HPC)

- *Where is it?* And in the case of pain – *Does it move anywhere?*
- How would they describe the pain? – sharp, stabbing, dull, aching, squeezing? (let them use their own words).
- Time course. *When did it start? How did it come on? Was it sudden or gradual? How did it continue? Did it come and go/ worsen/improve?*
- *Does anything make it better or worse?*

- *How bad is it?* Can they use a severity scale 1–10 or describe it in terms of how it affects their life?
- *Did you feel anything else?* First ask them an open question, then ask about specific symptoms that may also arise from the systems most associated with the presenting complaint.

At this stage you may have an idea of the cause. You may want to ask specific targeted questions to identify further evidence for your initial differential.

Past medical and surgical history (PMHx)

- *What medical problems do you suffer from currently and what problems have you suffered from in the past?* Find out, in particular, when were they first diagnosed.
- *How have you been recently?*
- *Have you had any surgery? When did this happen?*

Ask about important diseases that the patient may have forgotten to mention:

- Ischaemic heart disease (IHD), e.g. myocardial infarction (MI)
- Rheumatic fever
- Hypertension
- Diabetes
- Cerebrovascular accident (CVA)
- Pulmonary embolus (PE)
- Deep vein thrombosis (DVT)
- Asthma/COPD
- Epilepsy
- Jaundice
- Infectious conditions.

Drug history (DHx)

- *What medications are you currently on?*
- *What dose do you take?*

- *How many times a day do you take it/them and at what times of day?*
- *How do you take it/them?* (oral or injection etc.)
- *Have you any allergies?*

Ask if anything happens to them when they take the drug. Sometimes the patient may be intolerant to the medication. However, be aware of rashes, swelling and other signs of anaphylaxis.

Family history (FHx)

Ask – *Are there any diseases that run in your family?*

Drawing a family tree will help to illustrate this. Diseases to watch out for are heart disease, strokes, hypertension, diabetes, cancer and genetic conditions.

Social history (SHx)

- *Do you smoke? Have you ever smoked for a significant period of time? When did you stop?*
- *How much do you/did you smoke on average every day?*

Express smoking as pack years. Number of years the patient has smoked, multiplied by the number of packs smoked per day. There are usually 20 cigarettes in a pack.

- *How much alcohol do you drink in an average week?* (express in units)
- *What do you do for a living?*
- *Do you have any pets?*
- *Have you travelled anywhere recently?*
- *What sort of housing do you live in?*
- *Do you live with anyone else at home?*

Determine if they live alone in a house, flat, sheltered housing, residential or nursing home:

- *How are you coping at home?*
- *Are you able to cook/clean/wash/go shopping on your own or do you need help?*
- *Do you need help to move around?*
- *Do you need a walking stick/wheelchair?*
- *Do you have stairs to climb?*
- *Do you have any carers? How often do they come?*

Systemic enquiry (S/E)

At this stage, in order to conclude the history, it is important to ask about symptoms from systems not yet enquired about in the history of the presenting complaint (HPC):

- **General**: fever, weight loss, loss of appetite, lethargy
- **Cardiovascular system**: chest pain, palpitations, shortness of breath, paroxysmal nocturnal dyspnoea (sudden breathlessness during the night), orthopnoea (breathlessness on lying flat), leg swelling, nausea, sweating, dizziness, loss of consciousness
- **Respiratory system**: shortness of breath, cough, haemoptysis, wheeze, chest pain
- **Gastrointestinal system**: nausea and vomiting, haematemesis, dysphagia, heartburn, jaundice, abdominal pain, change in bowel habit, rectal bleeding, tenesmus (sensation of incomplete bowel emptying)
- **Genito-urinary system**: dysuria (pain on passing urine), frequency, terminal dribbling, urethral discharge
- **Gynaecological system**: pelvic pain, vaginal bleeding, vaginal discharge, LMP
- **Neurological system**: headaches, dizziness, loss of consciousness, fits, faints, funny turns, numbness, tingling, weakness, problems speaking, change in vision.

Although one can use the generalised template to obtain an adequate history, we have provided a range of questions, which will be useful when addressing different symptoms.

We have grouped the symptoms according to which physio-logical system they best represent, although some symptoms may belong to more than one.

CARDIOVASCULAR HISTORY

Chest pain

When taking a history of chest pain ask the patient:
- *Where is the pain?*
- *Does it move anywhere?*
- *When did it start and was it a sudden or gradual onset? What were you doing at the time?*
- *Since the onset, how has the pain continued – i.e. constant or coming and going?*
- *Can you describe its character?*
- *Does anything make it better or worse?*
- *Can you grade its severity from 1 to 10?* (1 is the least and 10 is the most).

◉ Target questions

Do you: suffer from hypertension, diabetes, high cholesterol? Have you ever smoked? Do you have any family history of heart problems such as angina or heart attack? **Risk factors for ischaemic heart disease (IHD)**

Does it hurt more on deep breathing or coughing, i.e. pleuritic chest pain? **PE, pneumonia**

Do you have a fever or a productive cough? **Pneumonia**

Recent surgery, recent immobility – long haul flights, bed rest, on the pill/HRT, current diagnosis of cancer, previously diagnosed PE/DVT, pro-clotting disorder, swollen tender legs? **PE risk factors**

Have you done any recent straining/lifting? **Musculoskeletal/IHD**

Do you have any history of heartburn, hiatus hernia or reflux disease? **Gastro-oesophageal reflux disease (GORD)**.

Palpitations

When taking a history of palpitations ask the patient:

- *When did you first notice palpitations?*
- *Do they occur continuously or do they come and go (paroxysmal)?*
- *Were they fast or slow? Were they regular or irregular? Did you notice extra beats? Can you tap the beat with your hand?*
- *What were you doing at the time?*
- *Did you experience any other symptoms such as chest pain, shortness of breath, loss of consciousness/feeling faint, leg swelling?*

◉ Target questions

Were you very anxious? **Anxiety provoked**

Do you have a fever? What medications are you taking? **Sinus tachycardia**

Do you have any heart murmurs or valve problems? Do you have any thyroid problems? Do you suffer from angina? Have you had a heart attack? How much alcohol do you drink? **Atrial fibrillation**

Shortness of breath – see *Respiratory history*, below

Loss of consciousness – see *Neurological history*, p. 75.

RESPIRATORY HISTORY

Shortness of breath

When taking a history of shortness of breath, ask the patient:

- *How long have you been short of breath?*
- *Do you normally get short of breath?*

- *Has it got worse recently?*
- *Did it come on suddenly or gradually?*
- *What were you doing at the time?*
- *Is there anything that makes it better or worse?*
- *How far can you walk before having to stop due to breathlessness?*
- *Do you get short of breath on lying flat? How many pillows do you sleep on?*
- *Do you ever wake up in the middle of the night feeling breathless?*

◉ Target questions

Do you cough up anything? What colour is it? Do you have chest pain which is worse on breathing in deeply? **Lower respiratory tract infection (LRTI)**

Do you get short of breath when lying flat or in the middle of the night? Have you noticed your legs getting more swollen? Do you have any known heart problems? Are you taking any water tablets (diuretics)? Are you good at taking them? **Left ventricular failure**

How much do you smoke? Have you been gradually getting more breathless for a while? Do you cough up phlegm most of the time? **Chronic obstructive pulmonary disease (COPD) or infective exacerbation**

Do you have sharp chest pain that is worse when you breathe in? Do you have tender swollen legs? Have you coughed up any blood? Check if there are any other PE risk factors – recent surgery, recent immobility, long haul flights, bed rest, on the pill/HRT, current diagnosis of cancer, previously diagnosed PE/DVT, pro-clotting disorder. **Pulmonary embolus (PE)**

Do you suffer from or have a family history of asthma, eczema, hay fever or allergies? Is it worse at night or in the morning? Does exercise, cold air or pollen make it worse? Do you get heartburn? **Asthma**

Have you had any recent chest injury or trauma? **Pneumothorax**

Have you noticed any tingling? Swollen lips? Rash? Have you any allergies? **Anaphylaxis**

How is your appetite? Have you noticed any weight loss? Do you feel tired? How much do you or have you smoked? **Bronchial cancer**

Cough

When taking a history of a cough, ask the patient:
- *How long have you been coughing for?*
- *Do you bring anything up? What colour is it?*
- *When do you cough? Does anything make it better or worse?*
- *Have you noticed any blood in your sputum?*

⊙ Target questions

Do you cough up yellow/green sputum? Are you short of breath? Have you any chest pain? Fever? Any recent travel? Do you have any pets? **LRTI**

Do you have any history of heart problems? Do you have swollen ankles, get breathless lying flat or wake up in the middle of the night feeling breathless? **Left ventricular failure**

Do you suffer from or have a family history of asthma, eczema, hay fever or allergies? Is it worse at night or in the morning? Does exercise, cold air or pollen make it worse? Do you get heartburn? **Asthma**

Have you coughed up any blood? Do you have sharp chest pain that is worse when you breathe in? Do you have tender swollen legs? Check on any other PE risk factors – recent surgery or recent immobility, long haul flights, bed rest, on the pill/HRT, current diagnosis of cancer, previously diagnosed PE/DVT, clotting disorder. **PE**

How is your appetite? Have you noticed any weight loss? Do you feel tired? How much do you, or have you smoked? **Bronchial cancer**

Have you started any new medications, e.g. **ACE (angiotensin-converting enzyme) inhibitors**

Do you have a runny nose? **Post-nasal drip**

Wheeze

When taking a history of a wheeze, ask the patient:
- *How long have you been wheezy for?*
- *Do you get it all the time or only intermittently?*
- *Do you get short of breath?*
- *Is there any chest pain?*
- *Do you have a cough?*

◉ Target questions

Do you suffer from or have a family history of asthma, eczema, hay fever or allergies? Is it worse at night or in the morning? Does exercise, cold air or pollen make it worse? Do you get heartburn? **Asthma**

How much do you smoke? Have you been gradually getting more breathless for a while? Have you coughed up phlegm most days, for more than 3 months? For more than 2 years? **COPD**

Do you have any history of heart problems? Do you have swollen ankles, get breathless lying flat or wake up in the middle of the night feeling breathless? **Left ventricular failure**

Have you noticed any tingling? Swollen lips? Rash? Have you any allergies? **Anaphylaxis**

Chest pain – see *Cardiovascular history*, p. 61.

GASTROINTESTINAL HISTORY

Dysphagia

When taking a history of dysphagia (difficulty swallowing) ask the patient:

- *What have you found most difficult to swallow? Solids or liquids, or both?*
- *Where does the food stick?*
- *When did you first notice this?*
- *Did it come on suddenly one day or has it been a gradual process?*
- *When does it happen?*
- *Do you find it is painful to swallow?* (odynophagia)
- *Has food ever gone down the wrong way?*
- *Do you have a cough or feel short of breath?*

◉ Target questions

Has there been a gradual problem with solids or liquids? How is your appetite? Have you lost any weight? Do you smoke? Drink alcohol? **Oesophageal malignancy**

Do you find your swallowing problems come only every so often? Do you suffer from heartburn? Do you have problems drinking hot drinks? **Gastro-oesophageal reflux disease (GORD)**

Do you find your swallowing gets worse over the course of the day and towards the end of the meal? Do you become more physically tired and weak over the course of the day? **Myasthenia gravis**

Do you find the skin over your fingers and lips is tight? Do your fingers get cold, painful and change colour? **Systemic sclerosis**

Does it happen only intermittently? **Oesophageal spasm**

Do you gurgle when drinking? **Pharyngeal pouch**

Are you on iron tablets? **Plummer – Vinson syndrome**

Haematemesis

When taking a history of haematemesis (blood in vomit), ask the patient:

- *When did it start?*
- *Was this of sudden onset or have there been previous smaller episodes?*
- *How much blood did you vomit?*
- *Is it fresh blood or clotted blood? Does it look like coffee grounds?*

◉ Target questions

Were you retching or vomiting before the blood? **Mallory – Weiss tear**

Do you have pain in your upper abdomen? Do you have any past history of indigestion or ulcer disease? **Ulcer bleed**

Are you on painkillers or blood-thinning drugs? **Gastritis from NSAIDs, aspirin, warfarin**

Do you drink alcohol and how much? Have you any liver problems? **Variceal bleed**

Have you noticed any weight loss or decreased appetite? Any problems swallowing? **Upper GI cancer**

Is the stool black in colour? **Melaena**

Diarrhoea

When taking a history of diarrhoea, ask the patient:

- *How long have you had it for? Longer than 2 weeks?*
- *When was the last formed stool that you passed?*
- *What is the consistency of the stool?*
- *How often do you pass stool? How much stool do you pass?*
- *Have you noticed any blood in your stool?*
- *Do you get this regularly?*
- *Have you been previously investigated for this?*

⊙ Target questions

Do you suffer from fevers, abdominal pain or vomiting? Have you eaten any uncooked foods? Have you travelled anywhere recently? Is anyone else you know affected? Is it improving? Have you had it for less than 2 weeks? **Infective gastroenteritis**

Do you have blood in your diarrhoea? Do you have abdominal pain? Do you have mouth ulcers? Do you have a family history of inflammatory bowel disease? **Inflammatory bowel disease**

Have you lost weight? Have you had any loss of appetite? Do you have alternating constipation and diarrhoea? Do you have the feeling of not completely emptying your bowels? Have you had it for more than 2 weeks? **Colonic carcinoma**

Do you find your stool floats and has a greasy appearance? **Malabsorption, e.g. pancreatic insufficiency/coeliac disease**

Do certain foods seem to cause the diarrhoea more than others? **Coeliac disease**

Have you recently taken antibiotics? **Antibiotic induced**

Are you on laxatives? **Laxative abuse**

Are you diabetic? **Autonomic neuropathy**

Have you any thyroid problems? Do you feel hot and shaky? Do you find your appetite increased? **Thyrotoxicosis**

Jaundice

When taking a history of jaundice, ask the patient:

- *When did you first notice the yellow tinge to your skin and eyes?*
- *Have you ever had this before?*

⦿ Target questions

Have you any family history of jaundice? What medications have you been taking? **Prehepatic, e.g. Gilbert's syndrome**

How much alcohol do you drink? What medications are you on? Have you had any recent blood transfusions? Where have you travelled recently? Have you had unprotected sex recently? Do you inject intravenous drugs? Have you eaten any shellfish? Do you have any tattoos? Have you been in contact with someone with jaundice? **Hepatic, e.g. viruses**

Have you noticed any change in the colour of your urine or stool? Are you itchy? Do you feel bloated? Do you have any abdominal pain? Have you any history of gallstones? Have you had any weight loss or loss of appetite? **Posthepatic, e.g. cholangiocarcinoma, pancreatic carcinoma**

Rectal bleed

When taking a history of a rectal bleed, ask the patient:

- *When did you first notice the bleeding?*
- *What colour is it?* (bright red, dark; see p. 67)
- *Where did you notice it?* (on the paper, in the pan, mixed with the stool or covering the stool)
- *How much blood would you estimate it to be?* (thimble, cup or bowl full)
- *Is it with every bowel motion?*
- *Have you noticed any mucus?*
- *Do you have pain on passing stool?*

⦿ Target questions

Have you noticed a recent change in bowel habit? Do you have a feeling of incompletely emptying your bowels? How is your appetite? Have you noticed any weight loss? **Bowel cancer**

Is the blood bright red? Is your bottom itchy? Do you have haemorrhoids? **Haemorrhoids**

Is it so painful to pass stool that you do not want to? **Anal fissure**

Do you have diarrhoea, crampy abdominal pain, fever, an eye problem, joint pains, ulcers or weight loss? **Inflammatory bowel disease**

Are you known to have diverticular disease? Do you have a change in bowel habit, left-sided abdominal pain relieved by passing stool, or flatulence? **Diverticular disease**

GENITO-URINARY HISTORY

Haematuria

When taking a history of haematuria (blood in the urine), ask the patient:

- *What colour is your urine?*
- *Is it pure blood or mixed with urine?*
- *Are there any clots?*
- *Does it happen all the time when you pass water?*
- *How long has this happened for?*
- *Is it near the beginning, end or during the entire urine stream?*

◉ Target questions

Are you taking rifampicin? Have you eaten beetroot? (These cause discoloured urine.)

Have you had a fever? Stinging while passing water? Smelly urine? Lower abdominal pain or loin pain? Do you find you go to toilet more often during the day? Or at night? **Urinary tract infection**

Have you ever suffered from kidney stones? Do you suffer from pain in the loin or groin? Is there pain specifically in the lower tummy or genital area? Does the pain come in waves? **Kidney stones**

Do you feel tired? Do you have night sweats? Have you noticed any weight loss? Pain in your side? **Kidney or ureteric cancer**

Do you smoke? Have you been exposed to industrial chemicals, e.g. aniline dyes? Are you taking any medication, e.g. cyclophosphamide? **Bladder tumours**

Do you get up to go to pass urine often? Is it painless? **Prostatic cancer in men**

OBSTETRIC, GYNAECOLOGICAL AND SEXUAL HISTORY

The history should follow the same format as the general structure outlined in the *General history taking* section, p. 57, but the following added questions should be asked.

Past gynaecological history

- *Have you had any problems with your uterus, ovaries or vagina?*
- *Have you ever had any gynaecological surgery?*
- *When was your last cervical smear? What was the result?*

Past obstetric history

- *Do you have children? Have you had any terminations or miscarriages?*
- *Were the pregnancies to term?*
- *What was the delivery method?*
- *Were there any complications during the pregnancy, e.g. bleeding or infection?*
- *What were the birth weights?*
- *Were there any complications after delivery, e.g. depression?*

Menstrual history

- *When was the first day of your last period?*
- *Is your period usually regular? What is the cycle length? When did you start/stop your periods?*
- *Are they particularly heavy?* Ask about number of tampons or pads used, if clots or flooding occurs.
- *Do you suffer pain during periods?*

Systemic enquiry

- *Do you have bleeding in between your periods? After sexual intercourse? Since your menopause?*
- *How heavy is the bleeding? How many tampons or towels do you use? Do you have clots or find the bleeding is more than the pad or tampon can absorb (flooding)?*
- *Do you have vaginal discharge? What colour is it? How much is it?*
- *Do you suffer from pelvic pain? Do you have pain during intercourse? Is it superficial or deep pain?*
- *Do you wet yourself? Do you find you go to pass urine often?* Urinary symptoms can indicate gynaecological pathology.

Sexual history

This can be one of the trickiest histories because clinicians may get embarrassed talking about the sex lives of patients and do not wish to embarrass the patient. This history is not commonly used except in sexual health clinics, but it is important to know the questions that should be asked to be able to give a good differential diagnosis.

Apart from a GU clinic setting, the history will almost always be asked as part of another history such as an obstetric and gynaecological history. This means that the rapport with the patient has already been built up, so it is now very important to signpost your new line of questioning. This would be particularly relevant when considering a sexual condition in a non-sexual context, e.g. septic arthritis.

Start with – *You've just mentioned that you were suffering from problems with your genital area, and I would like to ask you further questions regarding this. The questions will be very personal, but please don't feel embarrassed and you don't have to answer them if you do not wish to. The questions are from a standard list that we ask all patients.*

Now use the history structure. People commonly present with:

- discharge
- itchiness
- sores and lumps.

The key questions to ask to ascertain risk to the patient and their partner are:

- *Are you sexually active?*
- *When the symptoms came on, was the person you had sex with a regular or casual partner?*
- *How many partners have you had in the past year?*
- *Were they exclusively male or exclusively female or both?*
- *Do you use sex toys?*

And for each partner, you should ask:

- *Were they a regular/casual partner?*
- *Did you have vaginal/anal/oral sex with them?* (With anal intercourse, it is important to know if they received it or were giving it.)
- *Did you use protection? What protection did you use?*
- *Did you pay the partner for sex and have you ever paid for sex?*
- *Did your partner at the time have a sexually transmitted disease?*

In this history, it is also important to ascertain HIV risk as well. You must warn the patient that these questions relate to this by saying – *Thank you for answering the questions truthfully, but I must also ask you some standard questions regarding the level of risk for HIV infection. Once again you don't have to answer these, but it would greatly assist my understanding of your problem if you did.*

Other questions relating to the risk of HIV infection:

- Sexual practices as above.
- *Have you ever injected drugs into your veins or have you had a partner or friends who have?*
- *Have you ever had a blood transfusion either in the UK before 1985 or abroad at any time? Have you been diagnosed with a blood disorder?*

Legal Guidance – Termination of pregnancy

The law governing termination of pregnancy has its roots in the 1939 case of R-v-Bourne [(1939) 1 KB 687, (1938) 3 All ER 615].

Mr Bourne openly performed an abortion on a 15-year-old girl who was pregnant following a rape. He was charged with a criminal offence but acquitted after the court decided that abortion was not illegal if it was performed because a woman's health – physical and/or mental – was in jeopardy.

This principle was eventually codified in the Abortion Act 1967. This Act was amended by the Human Fertilisation and Embryology Act 1990 s.37. Prior to the 1967 Act, abortion was a crime under common law in Scotland and under the Offences Against the Person Act 1861 in England and Wales.

The position now is that terminations of pregnancy are lawful, or to put it another way, that no-one will be guilty of a criminal offence if:

- the termination is carried out by a registered medical practitioner; **and**

- two registered medical practitioners have decided that the continued pregnancy would present a greater risk than a termination, in terms of the woman's physical or mental health, or that of any children she already has; **and**
- the termination takes place before the end of the 24th week of pregnancy.

Alternatively, a termination may be carried out by a registered medical practitioner without fear of prosecution, *without* time limit and *without* a second opinion where:

- there is a risk of grave permanent injury to the woman **or**
- the risk to life of continuing the pregnancy outweighs the risk of termination.

Or it may be carried out by a registered medical practitioner *without* time limit but *with* a second opinion where:

- there is a substantial risk that the child, if born, would suffer from severe physical or mental handicap.

Note: In emergency situations a second doctor is not required.

Conscientious objections

If termination of pregnancy conflicts with a doctor's religious or moral beliefs, they may be excused from performing the procedure. This exemption does not apply in emergency situations.

A conscientious objector must, however, explain their position to the patient and make arrangements for them to see another practitioner without delay.

NEUROLOGICAL HISTORY

Loss of consciousness

- *Was it witnessed?* Try to get answers from a witness.
- *When did this happen?*

- *What happened beforehand?*
- *Did you know you were going to lose consciousness?*
- *How long were you unconscious for?*
- *Did you hurt yourself? Did you hit your head?*

◉ Target questions

What were you doing at the time?

- Were you watching TV or flashing lights? **Epileptic fit**
- Were you coughing? **Cough syncope**
- Were you passing urine? **Micturition syncope**
- Were you turning your head? **Carotid hypersensitivity**
- Were you standing up? **Postural hypotension**
- Were you exerting yourself, e.g. climbing stairs? **Cardiac valve abnormality**

Did you have a warning? Any palpitations? **Arrhythmia**

Were there any visual or sensory changes? **Epileptic fit**

Did you wet yourself? Did you bite your tongue? **Epileptic fit**

How did you feel afterwards? Confused for a while? **Epileptic**

Did you feel fine afterwards? **Non-fit**

Did you feel weak or have muscle pain after coming round? **Epileptic fit**

Ask any witnesses what the patient looked like when they were coming round.

Headache

- *When did you first notice it?*
- *What were you doing before it started?*
- *Did you notice anything before the onset?*
- *How did it come on? Suddenly or gradually?*
- *How long has it lasted for?*

- *Where does it hurt?*
- *Have you ever had a similar one before? How often do they come on?*
- *How severe is it?* (Grade 1–10)

◉ Target questions

Was it the worst headache you have ever had? Did it feel as if someone had hit you on the head? Were you straining prior to onset? Was there any vomiting? Any neck stiffness? Any fear of lights? Is there anyone in the family who has had a subarachnoid bleed? **Subarachnoid haemorrhage**

Do you have a stiff neck? Fever? Dislike of lights? Do you have a rash or any joint pains? Have you been feeling unwell recently? **Meningitis**

Did you see any zigzag lines/other visual changes before onset? Was the pain mainly on one side? Did you feel sick or have you vomited? Did you want to go to quiet dark corner of your house? Has it been triggered by certain foods, e.g. cheese, caffeine or alcohol? **Migraine**

Does your headache occur frequently for a few weeks then stop for months in a cycle? Does it start around the eye and remain on that side of the head? Do you notice anything that might trigger it? **Cluster headaches**

Have you noticed any weakness or change in sensation? Is it worse on lying down? Do you feel sick? Have you vomited? **Raised intracranial pressure**

Have you recently stopped/started taking painkillers? **Rebound headache/analgesia induced**

Is your scalp sore? Does your jaw hurt after you have chewed for a while? Have you had any sudden loss of vision? Do you feel tired? **Giant cell arteritis**

Have you had any recent/current stresses? Does it feel like a general tightness around the head? **Tension headache**

Have you had any recent increased lethargy or confusion over the last few days? Have you had a recent head injury? **Subdural haemorrhage**

PSYCHIATRIC HISTORY AND MENTAL HEALTH

A psychiatric history is different from the mental-state examination which determines the actual mental state of the patient at the time.

Start off with:

- name
- age
- how they were admitted (elective vs police)
- presenting complaint.

Changes in mood

- *Have you felt low recently?*
- *What did you enjoy doing before? Do you still enjoy doing those things?*
- *How is your sleep pattern? (early morning waking or sleeping in?)*
- *How is your appetite?*
- *Do you still feel like sex?*
- *How do you see the future?*

Deliberate self harm

- *Have you ever had thoughts about hurting yourself? Have you done so?*
- *Have you ever had thoughts about ending your own life?*
- *Did you leave a suicide note or try to tie up your affairs?*
- *What exactly did you do?*
- *Do you have any regrets that you did not succeed? Do you have any intention to go and do it again?*

If you suspect paranoid schizophrenia it is advisable at this stage to ask about Schneider's First Rank Symptoms.

Past psychiatric history

- *Have you had any mental health issues?*
- *Have you ever seen a psychiatrist or been admitted to a psychiatric hospital?*

Past medical history

- *What is your health like?*
- *What medical problems do you suffer from?*

Drug history

- *Are you taking any doctor prescribed medication at the moment? What is it?*
- *Are you allergic to anything?*

Recreational drug history

- *Have you ever taken any recreational drugs? Are you doing so now? What are you taking? How do you take it? How much do you take?*
- *Do you drink alcohol? How much do you drink in a typical week? Have you had any today?*
- *Do you smoke?*

Criminal history

- *Have you ever been in trouble with the police? Do you have a criminal record?*

Life history

Find out about the patient, starting from their early childhood all the way to the present day.

Early childhood:

- *What memories do you have of growing up?*
- *Do you have any brothers or sisters? How was your relationship with them?*
- *Were you adopted or fostered?*

Later childhood:

- *Did you make any friends?*
- *How did you find school?*

Adulthood:

- *Did you go to university? How did you find university?*
- *Have you ever had a job?*

Sexual and relationship history

- *Are you sexually active? When did you start?*
- *Do you have sexual relations with men or women or both?*
- *Are you in a relationship? Tell me about your relationships up till now.*

Note any mention of sexual abuse that surfaces in the interview.

Personality

- *What was your personality like before this current illness?*
- *How would you describe it now?*

Thoughts and beliefs

These usually reveal themselves during the interview and direct questioning may not reveal them. One way is to ask very general questions:

- *How do you view yourself?*
- *How do you view others around you?*

Current social history

- *Do you have a job?*
- *Where do you live? Is it a hostel or your own place?*
- *Do you live with any one?*
- *How are your relationships with your partner, your family and your friends?*
- *Have you ever been in trouble with the law?*

Family history

Particular emphasis should be on any psychiatric problems, deliberate self harm or substance abuse, e.g. *Has anyone in your family had mental health issues/tried to hurt themselves/taken recreational drugs?*

Legal Guidance – Mental health

Categories of mental health patient

There are three categories of mental health patient: formal, voluntary and informal.

Formal patients are those who have been 'sectioned' or detained under the Mental Health Act 1983. Whilst such patients may be deprived of their liberty and be subject to other restrictions on their rights, they also have rights of appeal and other statutory protection.

Voluntary patients are people who have mental capacity to make their own choices regarding their treatment and have chosen to receive treatment as an inpatient. They have exactly the same rights as someone receiving treatment for a physical illness (see *Dealing with potential self-discharging patients*, p. 46).

An **informal patient** is an inpatient who lacks capacity to make choices regarding treatment but is not actively trying to leave. In the case of Bournewood HL v. United Kingdom (2004) the European Court of Human Rights held that it was unlawful to hold such patients without ensuring they have similar rights to formal and voluntary patients. The Government addressed this gap in the law by amending the Mental Capacity Act 2005. These new provisions close the Bournewood gap.

Overview of the Mental Health Act 1983 (as amended by the Mental Health Act 2007)

The 1983 Mental Health Act had two aims: to give specific rights to patients who are, or appear to be, suffering from a **mental disorder**, whilst at the same time allowing for their compulsory detention and treatment.

A mental disorder is defined as follows: **any disorder or disability of the mind.**

This includes, but is not limited to:

- affective disorders, such as depression or bipolar disorder
- schizophrenia
- neurotic, stress-related and somatoform disorders
- organic mental disorders, such as dementia and delirium
- personality and behavioural changes brought on by brain injury
- personality disorders and mental and behavioural changes caused by substance and/or alcohol misuse
- eating disorders
- learning disorders (as long as there is attendant abnormally aggressive or seriously irresponsible conduct for s.3)
- autism.

Alcohol or substance misuse does not of itself constitute a disorder or disability of the mind.

Part II of the Mental Health Act deals with the compulsory admission to hospital for patients not involved in criminal proceedings.

Short-term compulsory powers can only be used if the individual is suffering from a mental disorder of a degree that warrants their detention in hospital for assessment, or assessment followed by treatment, and if the detention is thought to be necessary for the health and safety of the individual or for the protection of others.

Longer-term compulsory powers can only be used if the individual is suffering from a mental disorder of a degree that makes it appropriate to receive treatment in hospital. Appropriate treatment must be available and the circumstances must be such that the treatment can only be delivered in a hospital setting. Additionally, the detention must be necessary for the health and safety of the individual or for the protection of others.

Psychiatric personnel involved

Section 12 doctor

A section 12 doctor has particular experience in the treatment or diagnosis of mental disorder and has received special training in the Mental Health Act. One of the medical practitioners making an application for detention must be s.12 approved.

Approved Mental Health Practitioner (AMHP)

An AMHP is a social worker or other professional approved by a local Social Services authority to carry out certain functions under the Act, including making the application for detention (which will then be supported by two medical recommendations).

Responsible Clinician

This is the person with overall responsibility for a patient's care. They will not necessarily be a doctor, but must be an Approved Clinician.

Approved Clinician

This is a mental health professional who has received special training and is authorised to make certain decisions under the Act. Again, they need not be a doctor.

Nearest Relative

Section 26 of the Act determines the identity of an individual's **nearest relative**. In order of priority it is the individual's:

- husband or wife or partner in a civil partnership (unless the couple are permanently separated)
- son or daughter
- father or mother
- brother or sister
- grandparent
- grandchild
- uncle or aunt
- nephew or niece.

Out of the above, full blood relatives take precedence over half blood, and out of each pair, the elder of the two takes precedence.

If the individual's parents weren't married when he or she was born, the mother takes priority over the father, unless the father also has parental responsibility, in which case it is the elder of the two parents.

If the individual normally lives with a relative who acts as carer, or otherwise has a relative who acts as carer for them, that person goes top of the list.

If the individual and someone else have lived together as a couple for at least 6 months, that counts as husband or wife.

If the person at the top of the list is under 18 and is not the individual's husband, wife, civil partner or parent, they do not qualify.

Mental Health Act sections

Section 2

Section 2 allows for **admission for assessment** for a period of up to 28 days. The application is made by an Approved Mental Health Practitioner or the patient's nearest relative (defined in section 26 of the Act) and must be authorised by two doctors.

Section 3

Section 3 allows for **admission for treatment** for a period of up to 6 months, with an option to renew for another 6 months and thereafter for a year at a time. The application is made by the patient's nearest relative or an approved mental health practitioner and again must be authorised by two doctors.

Section 4

Section 4 allows for compulsory assessment in emergency circumstances for a period of up to 72 hours, with the application being made by the nearest relative or an approved mental health practitioner. However, only one doctor is needed to authorise the admission. The doctor must confirm that:

- the case is one of urgent necessity
- that waiting for a second doctor to confirm the need for a section 2 detention would cause an undesirable delay.

If a second medical certificate is provided within the 72-hour period the admission becomes a section 2 admission.

Section 5

Section 5(2) allows for **compulsory detention of patients already in hospital** for a period of up to 72 hours.

Under section 5(4) a mental health nurse has a **holding power** for up to 6 hours whereby he or she can prevent an inpatient from leaving pending the arrival of a doctor or Approved Clinician.

Section 136

Section 136 allows for the **removal and detention of a patient from a public place** to a place of safety for a period of up to 72 hours. The power is exercisable by a Police Officer.

Guardianship

Guardianship orders are a mechanism by which a patient over the age of 16 can be compelled to:

- live in a certain place
- attend certain places for work, training or medical treatment. The patient cannot, however, be made to receive treatment
- receive home visits from doctors or other professionals.

Part III

Part III of the Act covers patients who are involved in criminal proceedings.

Section 35 authorises a Crown or Magistrates' Court to **remand an accused in hospital rather than prison** so that a **medical report** regarding an accused person's mental condition can be prepared. The remand may be for a period of up to 28 days, renewable in blocks of 28 days to a maximum of 12 weeks.

Section 36 authorises a Crown or Magistrates' Court to **remand an accused person in hospital rather than prison for the purposes of treatment**. The remand may be for a period of up to 28 days, renewable in blocks of 28 days to a maximum of 12 weeks.

Section 37 authorises a Crown or Magistrates' Court to make **Hospital or Guardianship Orders** regarding a person convicted of an offence or, where the person was not convicted due his mental condition, where the Court is satisfied he committed the offence as charged. The order may be for a period of up to 6 months, renewable for a further 6 months and thereafter for a year at a time.

Mental health in Scotland

 After much consultation, the Scottish Parliament enacted the Mental Health (Care and Treatment) Act 2003. This Act contains all the provisions relating to compulsory measures for mental health care, as well as provisions concerning people who enter the mental health system through the criminal justice process. A range of measures for both compulsory treatment and support for people who are not the subject of any compulsory measure are covered by the Act.

PAEDIATRIC HISTORY

Taking a history of a child is similar to taking that of an adult, but there are a few more questions that need to be asked. Some sections already mentioned in the adult history-taking section need to be emphasised.

Presenting complaint

Gather information about the presenting complaint directly from the child if they are old enough, or direct from the carer, usually the parents or legal guardian.

Obtain the time line of the complaint as children's illnesses can fluctuate over time.

Past medical history

- *Were there any complications during pregnancy?*
- *Was the baby born at term? What was the mode of delivery? How much did the baby weigh? Were there any complications at birth?*
- *Have there been any operations, hospital admissions, medical problems, e.g. congenital heart disease, asthma, epilepsy, diabetes or genetic disease?*

Developmental history

- *Do you have any concerns about your child's development?*
- *Has she been reaching her milestones:*
  - *Gross and fine motor, language, social skills?*
  - *Does she look up at you and seem interested in her surroundings? Does she smile?*
  - *Can she walk/crawl/pull herself up? What age could she do that?*
  - *Does she play with other children yet?*
- *Manual dexterity:*
  - *Can she hold a pencil and use it?*
  - *Does she transfer things between hands or show a preference for one particular hand?*
  - *Does she ever pick anything up with her index finger and thumb or does she try to clasp everything?*
  - *When did she start using her index fingers and thumbs?*
- *Can she speak words yet? When could she do that? What can she say?*

Immunisation history

Check that the child's vaccinations are up to date. If not, ask why not.

Drug history

Ask if the child is taking any regular medication and if they have any allergies.

Family history

- *Who makes up your family?* or *What family members are there?*
- *Are there any medical problems running in the family?* (very important to draw a family tree).

If – and only if – you have a compelling reason to ask, inquire tactfully about consanguinity, e.g. *Have there been any relationships between members of your family that produced children?*

Asking questions here needs particular sensitivity. Ask whether the child is doing well at school, who looks after the child, who makes up the family unit, and what do the parents do.

Systemic enquiry

Older children who are able to articulate their problems may be asked the same questions as adults.

For younger children ask the carers about:

- general – appetite, fever, rashes, alertness, crying (are they pacifiable?)
- CVS – breathing, wheezing, looking blue, sweating
- respiration – breathing difficulties, coughing
- gastro – appetite, vomiting, diarrhoea, abdominal pain
- genito-urinary – number of wet nappies
- ear, nose and throat (ENT) – ear discharge, grasping of outer ear, runny nose, noisy breathing
- neurological – fits, walking gait.

PREOPERATION CLINIC

This is a common area for questions in medical student finals, since it tests whether you have ever been to a pre-operation clinic. Conducting a preoperative interview is a fundamental skill for the F1 foundation year. The patients seen are most often there for elective or minor surgery. Most will be treated as day cases and will go home either the following day or even the same day. It is extremely important that any risk factors that may affect a patient's safety are identified in advance.

Preoperative interview:

- Introduce yourself.
- Ask about the operation the patient is coming in for (so that they know and you know that they know).
- Inquire if the patient is happy to proceed with surgery.
- Take a quick history of symptoms (*When did it start?*) and check on symptoms between the last clinic appointment and now.

Past medical and surgical history

Ask about ischaemic heart disease, diabetes, lung disease, kidney disease, chronic infection, joint problems (especially neck problems, e.g. cervical spondylysis) and clotting problems leading to DVT or PE. Try to use non-scientific language, e.g. *Have you had a blood clot in your legs or lungs?*

Ask about previous general and local anaesthetic exposure and any reactions to either: ask – *Have you ever been put to sleep before?*

Drug history

Ask about:

- what medications the patient is taking/has taken recently and their doses, paying particular concern to anticoagulants

- allergies – especially to drugs, rubber, latex, plasters or dyes
- vaccination status, especially tetanus.

Social history

Ask about employment, smoking, drinking, recreational drugs and social support available after surgery (e.g. is there anyone to take them home?).

Family history

Ask about any medical problems that run through the family.

System review

Ask about any other symptoms that may indicate an infection, which may in turn mean that the operation has to be postponed.

Then:

- Examine the patient and the part of the body that is going to be operated on.
- If appropriate, request bloods, chest X-rays, ECGs and any further investigations as required.
- Again, ask if the patient is happy to proceed with surgery, but tell them that the surgeon will run through the operation information on the day of the surgery.
- Give them certain preoperative advice: *Have nothing to eat or drink from midnight before you come in* (if they are a day case).
- For medication: see local preoperative protocols.
- Give them postoperative advice.
- Address any concerns or questions.
- Wish them well and tell them that you'll see them when they come in.

HIV counselling

At the time of printing, HIV remains incurable. Because of the length of the illness and publicity associated with the infection, the disease has been put on a special footing, with significant effects on social and personal well-being. Incurability and its links to sex have led to the strong stigma experienced by HIV sufferers, despite recent attempts to increase awareness in the general public and society as a whole.

There are certain threads common to discussions about HIV testing. When counselling before an HIV test or when there is an HIV-positive result, it is mandatory to explain the possible consequences of HIV. One of the legal requirements of testing is that a patient is able to make a well-informed decision before giving consent for a test.

See Chapter 5, *Explaining disease X*, p. 107 for advice on the basic structure of explaining disease to patients.

HIV – THE BASICS

Epidemiology

HIV is a disease caused by a virus and is not AIDS. It is currently incurable, but, with medication, some people who have the disease can live long and relatively normal lives. It is transmitted through sexual contact, in blood and blood products, or from mother to baby. It is a disease very common in areas such as sub-Saharan Africa, but there are a rising number of cases in the western world. It is not a common disease, but because it is not curable and a main source of infection is sexual transmission, it has developed a very high profile.

Pathology

The HIV virus attacks the immune cells in the body, and over many years (10–20 years), the body's response to infection decreases to such a low level that many viruses, bacteria and fungi attack the body. This end stage is AIDS.

Clinical features

Within a few weeks of being infected, people may develop a severe flu-like illness caused by the body trying to fight off the infection. It is in this period that the body produces antibodies to fight HIV and so the patient tests positive for the HIV antibodies. Most people ignore this illness, thinking it is simply flu.

Many years may pass, with the infected individual feeling normal and not ill. The diagnosis is then often made when some of the rarer associated conditions develop, suggesting HIV infection.

Transmission

HIV is known to be transmitted via bodily fluids, e.g. vaginal fluids, semen and blood, and there is a minimal amount in saliva. It cannot be passed on by talking to someone, handshaking, sharing cutlery/cups or using the same toilet seat/shower facilities. The most common ways are via unprotected sex, especially unprotected anal sex, and intravenous drug users sharing needles with infected individuals. Blood transfusions were a cause before 1985 (often in haemophiliacs) before screening was introduced.

Health advice

It is a good idea to give health advice:

- Practising safe sex, through the use of a condom – or abstinence.
- If a patient is an intravenous drug user, suggest not sharing needles and offer information about signing up for a needle exchange programme.

- Travellers should take HIV prophylaxis (medication) to high-risk areas and ensure they are in contact with their country's embassy or consulate in case they require a blood transfusion whilst visiting such areas.

Diagnostic or further tests

The test for HIV is a simple blood test, which takes around 5 minutes. If blood is taken at the GP practice, there will be a permanent record in the notes. Advantages of this are that all clinicians will be aware of the HIV status and manage conditions appropriately. However, strong disadvantages include the fact that the record is permanent: all clinicians will know and if insurance companies or other bodies demand access to their records, it will not be possible to hide the information.

The test may also be taken at the genito-urinary medicine (GUM)/sexual health medicine clinic, where notes are held separately, and in some clinics a number is used to identify the patient rather than their name. Advantages of this include the ability to keep the HIV status separate from a patient's usual clinical notes. However, keeping HIV status distant from the main records means that clinicians cannot make a fully informed decision about the patient's management in the case that they are not told by the patient.

HIV test results

- Results will take around a week to come back; however, same day results are possible.
- The patient will need to come back personally for the results of the test, as clinics usually do not give the results over the phone. They can bring someone with them for the results.

- Normally the test is taken at around 3 months after an episode where patients think they've been exposed, and a repeat test is normally taken at 6 months as well.
- Very accurate results are achievable.

Prognosis

HIV is not curable at the moment; however, drugs are available that can boost the immune system. Most people can live symptom free for years and carry out their normal daily activities. However, AIDS is often unavoidable because the medication may become less effective over time due to HIV virus resistance. The medication does promote self-healing of the immune system but does not stop the spread of HIV and its gradual destruction of the immune system.

Follow-up

- HIV-positive patients will need to come in for regular medical checks to monitor the infection. These are to test how much virus is in the body and the level of white cells left. These are also used as an indicator to show if therapy should be started.
- The patient will be seen regularly by an HIV consultant, to keep an eye on how things are. They will decide with the patient whether anti-HIV therapy should be started.
- It is also a good idea to test for other viruses, namely hepatitis B and C, since they are often found at the same time. These viruses can be curable with modern therapy. If they do not have hepatitis, then it is a good idea to have vaccinations against common diseases including hepatitis B.

SOCIAL IMPACT OF HIV

Monetary issues

An HIV-positive diagnosis will immediately bar sufferers from any form of long-term financial loan: this includes mortgages and sizeable bank loans. It will immediately bar sufferers from some types of insurance cover, for example life insurance; however, some policies will cover the policy holder in the event of an illness that is not related to HIV.

Close contacts

Remember that the doctor's primary concern is for the patient and confidentiality. In all but exceptional circumstances, this will need to be maintained. The patient does not have to tell any other person. However, there is an ethical consideration for the patient to inform anyone who might be at risk, e.g. sexual contacts (it is best practice to try to engage the HIV patient in discussions regarding the rationale for informing contacts for screening purposes, for example).

The patient will need to educate people to whom they may be disclosing this news that common myths about HIV are almost invariably false. These include the perceived risk of picking up the virus from toilet seats/washing facilities, kissing (though deep kissing has a theoretical risk), sharing plates and cutlery, and handshakes. This will help break down barriers and gain acceptance within society. However, it is very difficult to avoid the stigma of the disease and alter public perception of the disease, but the situation is improving.

If a pregnant woman has HIV, it will put the baby at risk of contracting HIV. When a mother is HIV positive, it is advisable to perform a caesarean delivery, rather than vaginal delivery, and not to breast feed the baby.

Support networks

Good support networks are available, such as the Lighthouse Society and the Terence Higgins Trust, both of which provide a wide range of information regarding the disease and the possibility of meeting other sufferers of the disease.

PRE-HIV TEST COUNSELLING

Patients come for HIV testing for several reasons:
- Genuine exposure to a known HIV source.
- Possible HIV exposure as a result of high-risk activities with persons of unknown HIV status.
- They may be concerned with their own well-being and uninformed about HIV transmission.
- Requirement for work, insurance policies and visas.

When counselling a patient before an HIV test:
- Introduce yourself.
- Ask them why they want the test and explore reasons for their concern about exposure to HIV.
- Ask if they have any idea what their result would be.
- Explain HIV: medical and social issues and the nature of the test.
- Determine HIV risk at this stage (see *Sexual history*, p. 72).
- Explore how they would take the news of an HIV-positive result: would they be devastated or relieved?
- Ask them about the availability of a support network if and when they get the result – friends and family or partner.

- Re-confirm their intentions to go ahead with the test.
- Offer them leaflets/websites about HIV testing.
- Offer an appointment.
- Gain explicit and written consent.

GIVING HIV TEST RESULTS

HIV-negative test result

Some good guidelines for counselling patients with a negative result are:

- Introduce yourself.
- Refresh their memory of the test – that they had a blood test previously to detect the virus and that the results are back – *The test you had done at 3 months after your episode of risk did not detect any evidence of HIV. The test is 99.5% accurate, so it is extremely unlikely that you are HIV positive. However, for extra reassurance, we would like you to come back in another 3 months for a confirmatory test.*
- Emphasise that this does not mean that they should discontinue precautions to prevent infection, including the use of condoms on all sexual contact occasions.
- Inform them about the routes of transmission and preventative measures.
- Let them know that they do not have to declare this test to any institution or any firm.
- Offer any further support they may need.

HIV-positive test result

This is almost inevitably bad news. However, it is possible that a positive diagnosis will provide a certain relief (see *Breaking bad news*, p. 24). A good guideline for counselling patients with a positive result is:

- Introduce yourself.
- Ask them what they're expecting. Do they have any inkling if it is a positive or negative result? Do they understand what the test was checking for?
- Say – *Thank you for coming in – we have the results from the test back now. Unfortunately the blood has been shown to have the HIV in it. This means that you are HIV positive.*
- Wait for any emotional outpouring.
- Say – *I know that this diagnosis can be devastating news and I am sure you have a lot of questions regarding HIV. I would like to break down some common myths regarding this disease and answer any questions. Please take your time – we're in no hurry.*
- Explain the medical and social issues around HIV.
- Explain that it is impossible to establish the time of infection and duration of infection.
- Explain that testing is very accurate (99.5%) at 3 months after first exposure, increasing to 99.9% at 6 months. They will need to have another blood test in 3 months to re-confirm.

Legal Guidance – HIV and AIDS

Patients with HIV

- It is illegal to discriminate against anyone with HIV or AIDS.
- You must not treat such patients differently.
- Because you should be adopting safety measures with all patients, it will not be necessary to, for example, wear two pairs of gloves, and such behaviour will almost certainly cause offence.
- Disclosures without the patient's consent or against their wishes can only be made in exceptional circumstances,

where it can be justified in order to protect others. Always seek legal advice in this situation.

> Information about infection status should not be disclosed outside the immediate medical team without the patient's explicit consent. For this reason infection status should not be noted on the outside of a patient's records.
> This sort of disclosure should only be taken at consultant level and then with the benefit of legal advice.

Doctors with HIV

- Doctors who are HIV positive or who have AIDS **must** consult with their employer about their duties.
- Whilst it is illegal to discriminate against anyone with HIV/AIDS, a change of duties may be justified in order to minimise risk to patients. Doctors should never rely on their own self-assessment of their risk to others.
- Employers must have policies in place to ensure staff confidentiality.

5 Explaining disease X

EXPLAINING DISEASES

Explaining a disease process is a core skill for all doctors. It is very important to explain fully to help a patient's understanding. As with all preceding advice about talking with patients, remember to maintain your professionalism at all times. Below is a generic approach to explaining diseases to patients:

- Introduce yourself.
- Check the patient's current understanding and expectations.
- Start with a brief summary of the clinical events that have been happening, e.g. *You were admitted for fits, we performed several head scans and it seems that you are suffering from a condition called epilepsy…*
- Allow a pause to give the patient time to assimilate the words, but not necessarily to achieve full understanding.

Key details that then need to be addressed in the consultation:

- **Epidemiology**: Is it a rare or a common disease? Who suffers from it? Is there an ethnic or gender predisposition? What is the cause (genes vs pathogen)?
- **Pathology**: What is the basic mechanism of how the disease process works? (do not forget to use patient-friendly language)
- What are the **clinical features** of the disease?
- Are there any **diagnostic or further tests** that have to be performed?
- **Prognosis**: What is the prognosis of the disease? What is the disease spectrum? Is the patient at risk from any complications from the disease?
- **Management**:
  - How is the disease treated?

- Are there are any drugs that are needed? (If there are, go onto *Explaining drug Y*, p. 145 and *Explaining device Z*, p. 171).
  - Is surgery needed?
  - Are there are any lifestyle changes that have to be made?
- What is the role of the family and partner in supporting the patient?
- Are there any support groups or websites that are useful for the patient?
- Are there any leaflets they could have?
- If no active treatment is possible, you need to be able offer **palliative care options** – supportive therapy, specialist support services, etc.
- **Follow-up**: Will there be multidisciplinary support? Will blood tests/scans be needed regularly? Will the patient be followed up by a specialist? Will there be any need for vaccinations?
- **Social impact**: Is there going to be any consequence for employment, driving, financial situations or schooling? Will there be any consequences for any future children? Will the patient's contacts – family and friends – need prophylaxis medicine? (e.g. TB)
- Summarise and answer any questions. Allow the patient time to take in all this new information.

EXPLAINING ASTHMA

When dealing with a patient (or carer of a patient) who has been diagnosed with asthma:

- Introduce yourself.
- Check current understanding and expectations.
- Start with a brief summary – *You were admitted for breathing problems, which the medical team think could be asthma.*

Epidemiology

Asthma is a very common disease affecting people of all ages and both sexes. There is a possible genetic link: people with family histories of asthma, eczema, rhinitis and multiple allergies may be more likely to have generations of asthma sufferers. There is no exclusive cause of the disease, but it is thought that the airways of sufferers are more sensitive to air pollution compared to the normal population.

Pathology

The following information is more advanced and may be helpful to a patient with a good understanding of disease – *Allergens cause bronchoconstriction (narrowing of the airways of the lungs) resulting in reduced air flow and the wheeze typically heard and shortness of breath. The inflammatory reaction also stimulates other cells to produce mucus and the accumulation of the mucus in the airway worsens the symptoms.*

Clinical features

Sufferers intermittently have bouts of wheeze, coughing, shortness of breath and phlegm production, though not all at the same time. Typically it's worse in the early mornings. Typically, also, there are triggers that provoke asthma attacks, such as cold air, exercise, smoke and dust mites.

Emergency help

If you notice that you have become severely wheezy, short of breath, start becoming blue or verging on exhaustion, you must go to hospital for specialist treatment for a severe asthma attack.

Diagnostic and further testing

There is not one single diagnostic test for asthma. However, a combination of tests is available to back up the diagnosis. Something simple we can do is to give you a peak flow meter (see *Explaining peak flow meters*, p. 175). You use it twice a day for around 6 weeks, note in a diary the values you get on the peak flow meter and bring it back in. We can then review the control of your asthma.

Prognosis

The asthma symptom range is vast: some people have one attack every few years while some have several attacks a month. At the moment we don't know which category you're in. However, most asthma sufferers live long healthy lives.

Treatment

Asthma is treated with a combination of drugs and lifestyle changes. There are two types of drug: relievers, which relieve the symptoms during an asthma attack, and preventers, which prevent attacks (see *Explaining asthma medication*, p. 152, *Explaining peak flow meters*, p. 175, and *Explaining inhalers*, p. 177).

Lifestyle changes

If you smoke, we strongly advise that you should give up smoking. The people living in the same house as you should stop smoking in the house. Good cleanliness around the house, such as regular airing of bed covers and damp dusting, will remove dust mites.

There are many support groups available for further information, e.g. Asthma UK – www.asthma.org.uk/National Asthma Society.

Follow-up

Most of your asthma management can be done by your GP. However, should the attacks become more frequent and uncontrollable, then a specialist review may be needed. You can keep track of the asthma control with the peak flow meter. Your GP practice may also have a specialist nurse for asthma, who will be able to show you how to use the medication and the peak flow meter, and answer your questions about the disease. We recommend that you should get the flu vaccine every year from your GP, and a once-in-a-lifetime vaccine to protect against pneumococcus infection.

Social impact

You should tell your employer and your life insurance company of your new diagnosis. It may affect your job and any insurance policies you may have. The disease can be very disruptive for children (schooling and growth) and for adults (poor sleep).

At the end of the interview

Summarise and answer any questions they may have. Further reading:

- www.nice.org.uk for latest management guidelines
- Asthma UK – www.asthma.org.uk/National Asthma Society

EXPLAINING DEPRESSION

When explaining a diagnosis of depression to a patient:

- Introduce yourself.
- Start with a brief summary of the clinical events that have been happening.
- Check current understanding and expectations.

Remember that depressed patients may have difficulty concentrating, so you need to be more patient with them in the consultation to ensure their understanding.

Epidemiology

Depression is a very common condition, affecting people of all ages, ethnic groups and both sexes. It occurs in varying degrees and more women tend to suffer from depression than men.

It can be caused by triggers such as childbirth (postnatal depression), bereavement and medical conditions such as Parkinson's disease.

Pathology

It is believed that the condition is due to a lack of certain chemicals, such as serotonin and noradrenaline, in the brain, and this imbalance causes the depression.

The following information is more advanced and may be helpful to a patient with a good understanding of disease – *The brain's emotional centres are diffusely spread out in the brain, but it seems that areas such as the limbic, prefrontal and frontal cortex are mainly affected by depression. There are many types of neurotransmitter in the brain and two of the most influential are noradrenaline and serotonin. There seems to be an inhibitory process causing a lack of these two neurotransmitters in the brain, which leads to a depression of mood. Because of the interactions with the rest of the brain, it affects a person physically as well.*

Clinical features

People who are depressed have two sets of symptoms, one that affects the mind, and the other that affects the body. With regard to the mind, people who have a low mood don't find so much pleasure in what they do and have a negative view of themselves and the future. They may be more irritable towards others. Moderately to severely depressed people may have suicidal thoughts. They may have such a poor view of themselves that they believe they are worthless or that parts of their body are dead – and they may act on these thoughts (self-harm). Depressed people may have different coping mechanisms: they may start drinking more alcohol, wasting money, gambling or getting into debt, etc.

With regards to the body, depression manifests itself with poor appetite, weight loss (though weight gain is possible), poor sleeping habits (e.g. waking early in the morning) and finding it difficult to relax. Sufferers may have poor libido. In more uncommon cases, symptoms may be the reverse and sufferers may eat more, sleep excessively and gain weight.

Diagnostic tests

There aren't any scans or blood tests to prove depression. People are diagnosed by using a depression questionnaire with a tick box answering process for the symptoms that are experienced. This can assess and can grade the severity of the condition. There are several questionnaires that can be used to measure the severity of depression and we may ask you to fill in one shortly.

Prognosis

There is a huge variation in the spectrum of depression. Most depressed patients have a mild form. Roughly a third of people with depression get better, a third of people will remain depressed or have recurrent episodes, and a third will get worse, perhaps necessitating admission to hospital.

Treatment and lifestyle options

There are many ways of treating depression. Mild forms are often helped by a change of lifestyle, taking more exercise, changing social circle or job. There are many psychological therapies ranging from cognitive behavioural therapy to art and music therapies.

There are several types of medication available for depression, and they are aimed at addressing the imbalance of the brain chemicals. Antidepressant drugs typically take around 2 months to work and are reserved for moderate and severe cases of depression.

There are many support groups available such as – www. nhs.uk/depression, the Mental Health Foundation and MIND.

Follow-up

Depression is typically monitored in the GP surgery to ensure that it's not getting worse. There are emergency services at the hospital should you one day become particularly depressed. There are many and varied support groups that can offer you more practical ways to combat depression and a chance for you to talk to other sufferers.

Social impact

As mentioned earlier when talking about coping mechanisms, depressed people can lose their jobs, get themselves into debt, develop an alcohol problem or drug habits, damage relationships and go into a downward spiral. This is something that you should be aware of and seek appropriate help if it starts to occur.

EXPLAINING ANGINA

When explaining a diagnosis of angina to a patient:
- Introduce yourself.
- Check current understanding and expectations.
- Start with a brief summary of the clinical events that have been happening – *You were admitted for a recent bout of chest pain; we conducted some investigations and think the chest pain is probably originating from your heart. We think you have a condition called angina.*

Epidemiology

Angina is a very common condition, affecting mainly those over 50 years old in the western world. Men are more likely to suffer from the condition, though this evens out after women reach the menopause.

Pathology

Angina is a disease where the arteries supplying the heart are narrowed by fatty deposits laid down over many years. When the heart demands more oxygen, such as during exercise, the flow of oxygen through the arteries cannot keep up with demand, leading to chest pain, a form of heart muscle cramp. It is part of a wide spectrum of heart chest pain.

Clinical features

People describe it as a gripping chest pain, a band-like tightening or someone sitting on their chest. It may go down the left arm or up to the neck. It can be brought on by exercise, sudden emotion and physical stress, and even cold air. It will last for around 30 seconds, then will fade away as your heart stops beating so fast. You may feel nauseous or short of breath.

Emergency help

*The obvious worry is that one day it is possible that you may have a heart attack. You will know you are having a heart attack, rather than suffering from angina symptoms, if you feel sweaty, the pain doesn't go away when you rest, and it is not relieved by your spray. The pain may well be worse than your normal angina pain and not relieved by your spray. **If you think you are having a heart attack, call an ambulance as soon as possible**.*

Diagnostic and other tests

The most common test to diagnose angina is an exercise stress test, which gives a good indication of the severity of the condition. We also need to run some more tests to check out your blood sugar and cholesterol levels. You'll then be booked in with a heart specialist for an angiogram, which is a dye test to look directly at the arteries of the heart (see Explaining angiograms, p. 189).

115

When patients cannot do the physical exercise test, we may use an alternative test, known as a pharmacological stress test, which involves a scan of the heart.

Prognosis

Angina is seldom a condition on its own. Patients often have associated diabetes, high blood pressure and/or high cholesterol, and may suffer the complications of these individual diseases. Arteries in other organs may also be affected, and angina sufferers are at a risk from strokes and kidney damage in the future.

Treatment and lifestyle options

There are lifestyle changes you need to make. You should stop smoking (if you smoke), only drink alcohol in moderation, eat less fatty food, take more exercise and lose weight. Just losing weight will bring your blood pressure down and reduce your risk of heart attack and stroke. Your family can greatly help in this by monitoring what you consume and sharing the change of diet to support you. You should perform mainly aerobic exercise, so that you exert yourself but do not trigger angina. This could include exercises such as walking, gentle swimming or gentle exercise at the gym.

There is medication to relieve the angina pain: there is a spray that you should carry with you at all times. This spray is sprayed under your tongue to relieve the pain (see Explaining GTN spray, p. 172). You may need tablets to control your blood pressure and high cholesterol, and improve the blood flow to your heart. There is a wealth of information available from the British Heart Foundation and Heart UK.

Follow-up

A heart specialist will follow you up. There are also cardiac specialist nurses available who can give advice. At your general practice, you'll have regular follow-ups to check your heart. We also recommend that you have the flu vaccine once a year and a pneumococcal vaccine once in your lifetime.

Social impact

You should inform your employer, who may be able to give you a less physically demanding job. The Driver and Vehicle Licensing Agency (DVLA) will need to be informed of your angina. Based on the test results you have, they will make a decision about whether to withdraw your licence. Clearly, having an angina attack may be fatal to you and anyone else in or near the car. It does not necessarily result in permanent loss of your driving licence.

With regard to sexual activity, having artery disease is a known cause of impotence and care must be taken if you think about using Viagra, because of interactions between this drug and your heart drugs.

EXPLAINING OSTEOARTHRITIS

When explaining a diagnosis of osteoarthritis to a patient:

- Introduce yourself.
- Check understanding and expectations.
- Start with a brief summary of the clinical events that have been happening – You have been complaining about a severe pain in the knee. The scan revealed that you are suffering from osteoarthritis.

Epidemiology

Osteoarthritis (OA) is a condition where the joints lose their flexibility and smoothness over time. A normal joint has cartilage over the ends of the bones and plenty of fluid to keep the joint supple. Over time, the cartilage is worn down and the fluid becomes thicker and less abundant. These factors in combination cause the symptoms.

OA is a very common disease, which mainly affects the older population. There is no genetic link associated with OA and no *infective agent has been associated with it. It is generally due to wear and tear, and it is believed that the vast majority of people have some OA changes (on X-ray) in later life.*

Clinical features

Typically, there is a lot of joint pain, most often affecting the knees, hips and the lower spine (the weight-bearing joints). The hands are also affected, being the most heavily used limbs of the body, and bony nodules may develop at these joints. The pain is often sharp and worse on movement. However, after some time moving the joint, the pain commonly disappears. If you don't move the joint for a while, you will notice it go stiff and lock, and you may notice a grinding feeling when next moving the joint.

Diagnostic and other tests

Osteoarthritis is typically diagnosed on X-ray, where bone changes can be seen. The disease needs to be quite advanced to be seen on X-ray. Typically on the X-ray, there is loss of space between the two ends of the bone and the surfaces of the bones become rougher. Some blood tests may be needed to differentiate osteoarthritis from other types of arthritis. More detailed scans can be performed to reveal the extent of the arthritis.

Prognosis

Unfortunately, because it is a disease caused by the use of the joint over a long period of time, it will not generally improve over time. People with OA can suffer from deformity of the joints and, in severe cases, may need to have operations to replace joints.

Treatment and lifestyle changes

There is no cure for OA but the aim is to maintain function for as long as possible. The best advice is to lose weight and build up muscles around the joint. This will take the strain as the joint gets further worn down. To build up muscles, you can use a hydrotherapy pool or gentle weights at the gym. Regular gentle exercise, paradoxically, has been shown to slow the progress of the disease.

There is no drug that will control the disease. The only medication available is pain relief, and this is well known to bring much improvement to a patient's life. There are many complementary therapies that may also be useful.

A good agency for extra information is Arthritis Care UK.

Follow-up

There is a lot of multidisciplinary support; you will be seen by a physiotherapist regularly to review how you're walking and to suggest exercises. You will also be seen by an occupational therapist, who may suggest walking aids or improvements to your house. Unless your osteoarthritis deteriorates, it can be managed by your GP. You may need X-rays every few years to see how the joints are deteriorating.

Social impact

OA has been shown to limit a person's everyday functions, such as washing, getting dressed, walking, etc. Everyday activities will have to be adapted: for example you may have to make use of home delivery for shopping, make greater use of public transport or even change jobs. You may be able to claim government benefits if the osteoarthritis severely reduces your capacity.

EXPLAINING APPENDICITIS (SURGICAL CASE)

When explaining a diagnosis of appendicitis to a patient:

- Introduce yourself.
- Check understanding and expectations.

- Start with a brief summary of the clinical events that have been happening – *You came here complaining of lower right abdominal pain; we conducted some tests and we think you could be suffering from appendicitis.*

Epidemiology

Appendicitis is a condition where there is inflammation of the appendix. It is one of the commonest surgical conditions referred to the surgical team.

Pathology

The appendix is an appendage attached to the bowel. It does not have a role in humans. Typically, it is found in the lower right area of the abdomen. There isn't a single cause for inflammation, but it could be due to hormonal processes in the body or, more commonly, faeces becoming stuck in the appendix.

Clinical features

Most people complain of a central tummy pain, which moves to the lower right side. They often feel sick and may have problems with their urination. They may be feverish and have been vomiting.

Diagnostic and other tests

The diagnosis is made based on what you've told us and on the findings determined when examining you. Blood tests also support the diagnosis. A CT scan of the tummy may help in diagnosis if it is unclear. However, the only way to examine and remove a truly inflamed appendix is with surgery.

Prognosis

Without treatment, there is a strong risk that the appendix may burst (rupture), which will lead to a severe abdominal infection. With surgical treatment, most patients will make a full recovery and resume their lives normally.

Treatment

The most common treatment for this condition is surgery to remove the appendix. This can be done with keyhole surgery or a small cut made in the stomach wall to remove the appendix (see Explaining appendicectomy, p. 214).

Follow-up

You can go home after the surgery within a day or two, if there are no complications. Usually, you will have no further problems. Complications will delay your recovery time. After going home, the district nurse or your practice nurse can remove the stitches after 10 days.

The following information is more advanced and may be helpful to a patient with a good understanding of disease – *Because an appendicectomy is surgery on the bowel, adhesions can occur afterwards, where scar tissue can form between parts of the bowel and cause bowel obstruction. If this happens, you will feel sick and vomit, have intense abdominal pain, not be able pass faeces or gas. The treatment of adhesions depends on their severity; some get better with simple measures, but in some cases further surgery may be necessary.*

Social impact

Because you are having an operation, we normally recommend around 2 weeks off work after the surgery. You should avoid heavy strenuous activity immediately after the operation. If you do heavy manual work, you should have 4 weeks off work, or be able to do light duties in order to return to work.

EXPLAINING CYSTIC FIBROSIS (GENETIC CONDITION)

When explaining a diagnosis of cystic fibrosis to a patient or a patient's carers:

- Introduce yourself.
- Check understanding and expectations first.
- Start with a brief summary of the clinical events and tests that have been conducted – *Your child has been seen following recurrent infections and the associated abdominal pain. The tests suggest that he has cystic fibrosis.*

Allow a pause to enable the parents to assimilate the information before continuing.

Epidemiology

Cystic fibrosis (CF) is a common genetic disease affecting 7500–8000 people in the UK. CF has a genetic basis – both parents must carry the gene for CF, even though they may not suffer from it themselves. If the parents are not sufferers, they carry the recessive gene and the chance of them having an affected baby is 1 in 4, a factor to consider for any future children. The gene is common, affecting 4 in 100 people. There may also be a family history of CF. (Statistics in this section are from the Cystic Fibrosis Trust.)

Pathology

In CF, an excess amount of sticky mucus is produced, due to a defective gene. The mucus affects areas such as pancreas, lungs and bowel, and causes the symptoms of CF.

The following information is more advanced and may be helpful to a patient with a good understanding of disease – *The CF gene codes for a chloride ion channel and a defect means that not enough chloride can pass out, leading to an increased thickness of mucus. The build up and lack of expulsion of this mucus leads to local bacterial invasion and infection. The build up of mucus also means that it blocks the secretion of normal enzymes in different organs, such as the pancreas.*

Clinical features

Excess sticky mucus affects many organs in the body and causes multiple problems. Typically, problems are most pronounced in the lungs and lead to difficulty in breathing and recurrent chest infections. In the pancreas, it can cause poor absorption of nutrients, fat in particular. This can cause problems with regard to growth and overall development of the child.

Diagnostic and other tests

One way to confirm a diagnosis of CF is to take a blood sample and look at the DNA profile. This can definitively confirm a diagnosis of CF. Another diagnostic test is to look at the salts in the sweat: the sweat test. Other tests can be performed to assess the function of the lungs and pancreas at a later date.

Prognosis

There is no cure for CF; nevertheless, most patients live fulfilling lives, though shortened in duration. Patients live on average to their 30s or 40s. However, the average lifespan is always increasing as better treatments are developed. Because the mucus creates a persistent stress on the organs, other disorders develop. Damage to the pancreas can cause diabetes, and stress on the lungs causes recurrent infections and permanent structural damage. CF sufferers tend to be

123

shorter in stature, less well developed and less fertile than non-CF sufferers. However, they have normal intelligence.

Treatment

At home, parents can feed their children high-calorie diets to coun- teract the problems associated with reduced absorption of nutrients. Dietary supplements can also be added to replace any minerals and pancreatic enzymes not being effectively absorbed. To remove the mucus in the lungs, a technique called postural drainage and active chest physiotherapy can be performed, where the parent can literally bang and dislodge the mucus. This is performed several times a day, but as the child grows older, they can do it themselves.

Preventative antibiotics can be prescribed to reduce the frequency of chest infections. Annual flu vaccinations are required. There are new drugs that can help break down the mucus, which may be considered later.

A good source of further information is the Cystic Fibrosis Trust UK – www.cftrust.org.uk.

Follow-up

Because of the large number of organs affected, there is a multi- disciplinary approach to CF. It normally consists of child-specialist doctors, nurses, education specialists and physiotherapists. The team will look after your child to ensure steady growth and development, and to monitor how well both he and the rest of the family are coping with the CF.

Social impact

Having a CF child, with the care needs they require, can be chal- lenging to the most patient of parents. CF children need more care and attention. There's likely to be a period of readjustment for you and any other children. As your child grows older, there will be issues of school activities and possible prejudice from other children, to deal with. As mentioned earlier, there are implications for future children, so it's advisable to see a genetic counsellor if you are planning more children. We can put you in touch with a genetic counsellor.

A prenatal diagnostic test is now available to identify affected fetuses in the uterus. This is done by a process called chorionic villus sampling at 11 weeks of pregnancy.

Further reading and information

Cystic Fibrosis Trust UK – www.cftrust.org.uk.

EXPLAINING TYPE 1 DIABETES

When explaining a diagnosis of type 1 diabetes to a patient or patient's carer:

- Introduce yourself.
- Check understanding and expectations.
- Start with a brief summary, about the clinical events that have been happening – *You were admitted for general tiredness and recurrent infection. We found that you have high levels of sugar in your blood and this leads us to believe that you have diabetes.*

Your patient may be a young adult or teenager and you will need to give them special consideration (see *Communicating with young people (adolescents)*, p. 36).

Epidemiology

Early onset diabetes is a common condition, almost exclusively affecting children and young adults under the age of 30 years. It affects roughly half a million people in the UK. It accounts for approximately 1–2% of the number of people with diabetes; 4–5% of the total population will be affected by all types of diabetes. (Source – Diabetes UK.)

Pathology

The body requires insulin to lower raised blood sugar levels. Insulin is produced in an organ called the pancreas. In type 1 diabetes, the body attacks the pancreas, destroying the insulin-producing cells. As a result, the pancreas can no longer produce insulin. We don't know why the body attacks the pancreas or what triggers it. It has been conjectured that a virus infection may be part of the trigger.

Clinical features

Commonly, type 1 diabetes sufferers complain of going to the toilet often and of feeling very thirsty despite drinking large amounts of fluid. They may drink 4–5 litres a day: a normal person would drink around 3 litres a day. Diabetics may present more commonly with urinary tract infections or some more unusual infections. They may be acutely unwell with severe lethargy and marked loss of weight over a short period of time.

Diagnostic and future tests

The diagnosis of type 1 diabetes is made following a blood test result showing a high blood sugar (over 11 mmol/l). Regular monitoring of the sufferer's blood sugar levels, eyesight, kidney function and sensation in the feet will be required throughout life. The intervals for checks will vary, however.

Prognosis

Most diabetics with good sugar control lead healthy, normal lives. Prolonged poor blood sugar control can have a catastrophic effect on future health.

Poor blood sugar control will affect:

- *nerves in the body, leading to foot ulcers and reduced ability to walk*

- *eyes, leading to possible blindness*
- *kidneys, leading to kidney failure.*

Diabetes is also a risk factor for heart disease, causing an increased risk of stroke and heart attack.

Treatment

Two modes of treatment are available to diabetics: drugs and lifestyle changes. Type 1 diabetics usually use insulin injections (see Explaining insulin injector pens, *p.173). Diabetics have to monitor their own blood sugar levels with a special device.*

Emergency help

Taking insulin creates a risk of having a very low blood sugar and becoming hypoglycaemic (going hypo). This condition is serious because of the risk of brain injury. When experiencing hypoglycaemia, people say they feel distant and cold, lose concentration and may black out. The solution is to always carry something sweet, such as a chocolate bar or sweets to eat if you feel like this. Special sugar packs are available to buy.

Lifestyle changes

- *If you smoke, you should stop smoking.*
- *Take plenty of exercise.*
- *Watch your weight (insulin increases appetite).*
- *Follow a low-fat diet (cut down on junk food).*
- *Reduce sugar in your diet (cut down on chocolate, biscuits, sweets).*

A good source of information is Diabetes UK – www.diabetes.org.uk.

Follow-up

A diabetes specialist nurse and a specialist consultant, your local experts, will be available to provide advice and education. The nurse and GP will monitor your blood sugar level; however, you will need to test yourself regularly. We also conduct a special blood test called HbA1c, which gives a good indication of long-term blood sugar control.

You will need to come to the clinic for separate blood tests every 8–12 weeks. We can also measure your blood pressure and weight. An eye specialist will keep checking your eyes and we have chiropodists who will monitor your feet. A consultant will give you advice regarding your regime and will help if blood sugars become uncontrollable. You will need to have the flu vaccine once a year and a once-in-a-lifetime vaccine to protect against pneumococcal infection.

Social impact

Type 1 diabetes may affect schooling, causing problems with self image and peer relationships. Diabetes can affect driving – DVLA needs to be notified of your condition. You will not be able to drive until your blood sugars have stabilised, and you will need your eyes tested before your licence is re-issued. Your car insurance company may amend your car insurance premium.

For a young person, it may be difficult to implement dietary changes and this is where good family support comes in. If pregnancy occurs, there are also risks to the fetus and more support will be required during the antenatal period.

Further information

Diabetes UK – www.diabetes.org.uk.

EXPLAINING TYPE 2 DIABETES

When explaining a diagnosis of type 2 diabetes:
- Introduce yourself.
- Check understanding and expectations.
- Start with a brief summary of the clinical events that have been happening – *You were found to have repeated infections associated with long-standing tiredness. Blood tests*

showed that your blood sugars are raised and this means you have type 2 diabetes mellitus.

Epidemiology

Type 2 diabetes (also called non-insulin dependent diabetes) is very common and an ever-increasing problem Most people who suffer from the disease have a history of obesity, poor diet or lack of exercise. People from the south Asian continent, e.g. India, Bangladesh and Sri Lanka, are very prone to develop type 2 diabetes. It affects mainly the older population: people are most often diagnosed aged 40–60 years. There are an estimated 2 million sufferers in the UK. In recent years it has begun to affect young people who are obese. (Source – Diabetes UK.)

Pathology

The body requires insulin to control blood sugar levels. Insulin is produced in an organ called the pancreas. In type 2 diabetes, the body develops insulin resistance after years of high blood sugar levels, caused by poor diet, causing the cells of the body to become accustomed to high insulin levels. With the effectiveness of insulin reduced, blood sugar levels are not properly controlled and can become very high, causing the symptoms of type 2 diabetes.

Clinical features

People with type 2 diabetes complain of increasing tiredness; they might notice their vision going blurry, have a number of unresolved skin infections or have urinary infections. They might feel thirsty and dry despite drinking lots of water.

Diagnostic tests

For most patients, no further diagnostic tests are needed. In a small proportion of patients, a simple test (glucose tolerance test) involving drinking a known amount of sugar and testing the blood sugar level after 2 hours, will be definitive. Because diabetes is a risk factor for heart and kidney disease, we would like to test your blood for kidney function and cholesterol level, and measure your blood pressure, do a scan of your heart and check out your eyes and feet.

Prognosis

If you control your blood sugars well, you are less likely to develop the complications of diabetes. There is still an increased risk of stroke and heart attack. Poorly controlled diabetes can affect the peripheral nerves in your legs (causing ulcers on the feet), kidneys (leading to eventual kidney failure, which may require dialysis or transplantation) and eyesight (which may cause blindness).

Treatment and lifestyle changes

The first line of blood sugar control involves adjustments to the diet, which can be successful for a number of years.

The best diet:

- *is low in fat*
- *contains a good proportion of complex sugars (carbohydrate)*
- *should be one third protein (fish and meat).*

Should dietary changes fail, then tablets may help. We may also need to treat you for high blood pressure and cholesterol.

General lifestyle changes advised are joining a weight-loss programme, regular exercise of at least 30 minutes a day, giving up smoking and only drinking alcohol in moderation. These measures will also increase your blood sugar control and reduce the risk of heart attack and stroke. Good family support will help to overcome any difficulties adapting to the new regime.

A good source of information is Diabetes UK – www.diabetes. org.uk.

Follow-up

A diabetes specialist nurse and the local specialist doctor will be available to provide advice and education. The nurse and GP will monitor your blood sugar levels, but you can also test yourself two or three times a week. We also monitor the level of a marker in blood level called HbA1c, which is a good indicator of long-term blood sugar control. You will need to come in for blood tests every 12–16 weeks, when we can also measure your blood pressure and weight. An eye specialist will monitor your eyes, and a chiropodist will monitor your feet. A consultant will be notified; he will give you advice regarding your regime and will be available if your blood sugars become uncontrollable. There may be a specialist GP service in your local area. You will need to have the flu vaccine once a year and on one occasion the pneumococcal vaccine.

Social impact

Having diabetes affects many aspects of life. It affects long-term loans and mortgages, as well as insurance policies, such as health or travel insurance. You must inform the DVLA of your diagnosis because of the risk to your eyesight. It may also affect your employment if changes are required for you to stay in the same job, or another role may have to be found. Some occupations are not available to those who have diabetes. However, well-controlled type 2 diabetes need not disrupt your normal activities.

EXPLAINING HEPATITIS B

When explaining a diagnosis of hepatitis B to a patient:

- Introduce yourself.
- Check understanding and expectations.
- Start with a brief summary of the clinical events that have been happening – *You were admitted with tiredness and jaundice. The blood test shows that you have an infection of the liver called hepatitis B.*

Epidemiology

Hepatitis B is not a common condition in the UK. However, in areas such as south-east Asia, India and Africa there are large numbers of people with hepatitis B. Hepatitis B is a viral infection. It is commonly contracted through sexual contacts, intravenous drug use (sharing needles) or when an infected pregnant mother passes it to her children.

Pathology

When the virus enters the body, it triggers an immune response very much like flu. However, particles on the surface of the virus are difficult for the body to eradicate.

Prognosis

The most likely, but rare, complication of hepatitis B is that it reduces liver function and eventually causes liver failure by causing cirrhosis. However, cirrhosis is quite rare. Most patients eliminate the virus, but will have markers in their bodies showing that they were once infected. Even if you're unlucky and have a chronic hepatitis infection, there is a treatment regime available to remove the virus, but this would have to be done under specialist care. Having hepatitis B is also a risk factor for liver cancer.

Clinical features

Most people develop flu-like symptoms (shivers/chills/bone and muscle ache/fever) and their skin and the whites of their eyes may take on a yellow tinge. The flu-like symptoms subside in a few weeks, after which people can be symptom free for years.

Diagnosis and future tests

A simple blood test can confirm if the hepatitis B virus is present. You will need to be screened for other chronic liver diseases, such as hepatitis C. It is also highly advisable to have an HIV test.

Treatment

The most common treatment for hepatitis B is the use of simple drugs to reduce the temperature and relieve pain. This should be enough for the vast majority of patients. If you suffer from sudden bruising or nose bleeds, or suddenly take on a yellow tinge, you will need to be admitted urgently to hospital for treatment of possible liver failure. You should avoid all alcohol during active infection.

Lifestyle changes

If you're not a person with a chronic infection, there is no chance of passing on the infection. However, if you are unfortunate and develop chronic hepatitis, you will need to be aware that it is mainly transmitted via bodily fluids such as semen, vaginal fluids and blood. Care needs to be exercised in intimate situations. Using condoms for protection is a very useful way to prevent infection. If you're pregnant, the baby should be tested after birth.

A good source of information is the British Liver Trust.

Follow-up

All patients will see a liver specialist. If you have chronic infection, you'll need to have regular blood tests to check your liver function. A liver specialist is likely to regularly review you and organise a treatment regime. Your sexual partner will be offered a vaccine for hepatitis B.

Social impact

Hepatitis B affects long-term loans and policies such as life insurance and mortgages, especially if you're a chronic carrier of the virus, because of the risk of severe liver damage. There may also be stigma, because it is a sexually transmitted disease. You may be asked whether you would be willing to be involved in a programme to locate the source of the infection – this is called contact tracing.

133

EXPLAINING ECZEMA

When explaining a diagnosis of eczema to a patient or a patient's carer:

- Introduce yourself.
- Check their understanding and expectations.
- Start with a brief summary of the clinical events that have been happening – *You have attended with a skin condition. This is a form of eczema, which is a relapsing skin condition.*

Epidemiology

Atopic eczema is one of the most common skin conditions. It can affect anyone, but it has been shown that it can run in families that can have eczema traits. It is a condition associated with asthma, hay fever and other allergies. Families with these conditions are more likely to have members with eczema. However, no specific known cause is identified in the majority of individuals.

Pathology

There are triggers which can make eczema worse, such as cold air, dryness and perfumed cosmetics. In children it is occasionally associated with intolerance to cow's milk.

Clinical features

Typically, the skin at the knees, wrists, inner elbows and face becomes dry, then itchy. Patients tend to scratch at it, which can then cause local bleeding and even infection. Itchiness is the most irritating feature; it can keep people from doing their everyday activities and disturb their sleep. Unfortunately, eczema can cause prolonged scarring and may make the skin thickened and look older and more wrinkled. Other forms of eczema exist, e.g. in elderly people, which can affect the lower legs and feet. In babies and very young children, it can affect the whole body. The other major form of eczema is caused by long-term contact with substances, such as hair dyes, detergents and nickel, which cause a reaction. In these cases, it is easy to spot and diagnose, as the eczema is in the same places where contact with the irritant occurs.

Diagnostic tests

There is no diagnostic or confirmatory test for atopic eczema. However, because of the association with asthma and allergies, we would like to test you for any allergies. We will monitor you to see if asthma develops. Patch testing is available if specific triggers are suspected. Some causes may be identified through blood tests, e.g. milk allergy or nut allergy.

Prognosis

Nearly all eczema sufferers live normal healthy lives.

Treatment

The first line of treatment is simple moisturisers applied to the affected skin areas. Creams such as aqueous cream, when smeared on, have a very relieving effect. They need to be used very regularly. Soap substitutes are also used. If these don't work, then we can try steroid creams, starting at the mildest to reduce the inflammation. For children, a wet wrap technique is useful, whereby you can moisturise the skin in an easily managed way.

Lifestyle changes

It's a good idea not to be in cold conditions, but heated rooms should also not be too hot. So when you go to sleep, a hot wet towel on a radiator/humidifier can give enough moisture for a good night's sleep. Regular cleaning of bed linen has also been shown to help. It is *imperative, of course, to avoid the triggers. A good source of information is from the National Eczema Society – www.eczema.org.*

Follow-up

Eczema can be followed up in the GP clinic. If it starts becoming uncontrollable despite increasing medication, then a referral to a specialist may be necessary. No further blood tests or scans are needed.

Social impact

Eczema is a condition that can affect a person's work and their relationships, especially those with other children. Because it can affect the face, it can also affect self-confidence.

EXPLAINING EPILEPSY

When explaining a diagnosis of epilepsy to a patient:
- Introduce yourself.
- Check understanding and expectations.
- Start with a brief summary of the clinical events that have been happening – *You were admitted for fits, we performed several head scans and we believe that you are suffering from epilepsy.*

Epidemiology

Epilepsy is the one of the most common diseases affecting the brain. It affects roughly half a million people in the UK. (Source – National Society for Epilepsy.) *Both sexes and all races are affected equally. There is no known cause of epilepsy, though it may follow an infection of the brain or an injury to the brain. On very rare occasions, it can be the first sign of a tumour of the brain, which is why we did the head scans.*

Pathology

Doctors think that some people's brain cells tend to be more excitable than others, either naturally or via triggers such as head injury and infection, leading to seizures.

Features

Typically, people experience an aura, such as flashing lights, feeling numb, or a sense of déjà vu. They then lose control of what they can do. They may scream, thrash around, wet themselves or bite their tongue. Afterwards, they are sleepy and drowsy, and have no recollection of the event. Children sometimes suffer petit mal fits, where they lose their concentration and appear blank, as if in a trance. Fits can occur at any time, but common triggers include flashing lights and strobe lighting.

Diagnostic tests

You have had a scan of your head, which ruled out any disease of the brain. The diagnostic test was your brainwave test, the EEG, which showed an abnormality that is consistent with the pattern of fits you've been having. We have also completed other tests, which rule out other causes.

Prognosis

The experience of epilepsy is vast: some people will be fit free for years, have one fit, and then be fit free for many more years. Others have more frequent fits and need medication to control them. We will need to observe the pattern of the frequency of your fits to know more clearly which group you fall into.

Treatment

We do not generally start medication straight away. However, should the need for treatment arise, you will be duly counselled about it.

Lifestyle changes

We advise all patients:

- *not to swim alone*
- *not to lock toilet/bathroom doors*
- *to avoid triggering factors*
- *not to climb ladders.*

A good source of information is from the National Society for Epilepsy – www.epilepsynse.org.uk.

Follow-up

Epilepsy control can generally be managed with your GP's support. If the frequency of your fits worsens, then the GP will refer you to a neurologist for a review. You may need further scans and blood tests at intervals to assess drug levels to ensure they are adequate.

Social impact

Epilepsy will affect your ability to hold a driving licence and car insurance. The current rules are that you are banned from driving for 1 year automatically and you will need to be fit free for a minimum of 2 years before you can be considered fit for driving. The exception to this is when you have fits only at night during sleep.

Epilepsy may affect the type of work you can perform. You may have to change roles, for example if you operate heavy machinery. It will also affect premiums for things such as private health insurance. Being on epilepsy medication might well affect other medication you may need to take, e.g. the oral contraceptive pill or blood-thinning agents.

Further information and reading

National Society for Epilepsy – www.epilepsynse.org.uk.

EXPLAINING CANCER

A diagnosis of cancer, of whatever origin, will be devastating news to the patient. Worries about the future, metastatic spread, years of ill health, no certainty of cure, and the prospect of surgery or adjuvant therapy, make it a troubling diagnosis to live with.

The aim of this section is to provide a framework to explain any cancer, rather than a particular type. For F1 doctors/students, explaining a diagnosis of cancer is not routinely required, since any explanation will be plagued with statistics (e.g. rates of survival with no treatment or surgery etc.) and these statistics vary every year depending on research study and scientific progress.

Read *Breaking bad news*, p. 24 first.

Epidemiology

For a common cancer, you could say, for example – (use relevant cancer type here) *cancer is one of the most common cancers and especially affects those who smoke or drink* (or other relevant lifestyle/occupational trigger).

Pathology

Cancer originates from the cells of any tissue and the cause is unknown. However, certain risk factors have been identified, e.g. smoking, alcohol intake, using dyes and infectious diseases. Cancer is essentially damage to the cell's multiplying mechanism, so that the cells grow out of control, forming a tumour. As a result of its increasing size, the tumour can compress local structures or infiltrate nearby organs. The mass may itself ulcerate or bleed. A common occurrence is that the cancer spreads via the blood stream to other organs, e.g. bone and the liver.

Clinical features

The symptoms come from either the effects of the tumour growth on local structures or the structure itself. For example, stomach cancer can cause people to vomit blood. Those with cancer which has spread will also experience tiredness, weight loss and a sense of never being truly hungry. Bone cancer typically presents with unexplainable fractures to bones, bone pain and changes to the blood chemistry.

Prognosis

Prognosis depends on the route taken to treat the cancer, the type of tumour and how far it has spread. In general, the more widely the cancer has spread, the less good the prognosis, compared to a cancer in one area.

Diagnostic or further tests

The choice of investigation will depend on the location of the cancer. However, in almost all cases, a sample of the tumour should be taken for analysis. This analysis will show the type of tumour and, as a result, the best treatment can be identified. Typically, a patient will undergo scans of the area, e.g. CT. Sometimes, cancers can be examined with camera tests (endoscopy), where doctors can directly visualise the cancer and take samples from it.

Management

There are three main types of treatment. If the tumour is thought to be benign or low risk, doctors may have a 'watch and see' policy. With a more aggressive tumour, it is best to remove it if this is possible. This can be done by surgery; adjunctive chemotherapy or radio therapy can be used to shrink the tumour prior to surgery. These interventions are not without side effects and will not be considered lightly. Despite the best intentions, there are cases where such interventions do not work.

Cancer in the UK is treated using a multidisciplinary approach – the team includes: the cancer specialist, the surgeon, the GP, specialist nurses and dieticians. They will closely monitor your therapy and your health.

Follow-up

All cancers are followed up using the multidisciplinary approach, to check whether the cancer comes back after treatment or becomes larger and spreads. More tests will almost certainly have to be performed; these may be blood tests or scans etc. After a period of surveillance, which is likely to be years, the cancer specialist may eventually discharge you from their care.

For many types of cancer, there are dedicated websites, as well as support groups set up and run by previous sufferers. They are a great way to ask questions and share experiences with other patients.

Social impact

The diagnosis of cancer is certainly devastating for the patient and also for those close to them. It leads to a period of uncertainty and readjustment for all parties concerned and it can be emotionally draining. It is important that family members support each other during this time and do not become divided because of it. A key role for the clinical team is to provide this support.

Explaining drug Y

HOW TO EXPLAIN ANY MEDICATION

Explaining a new medication to a patient is another key skill a doctor must have. A patient's full understanding of a drug will increase the likelihood of their sticking to the regime and allowing the medication to demonstrate its full effect. Either new drugs are being prescribed, because they are being started for a new disease, e.g. antibiotics for an infection, or old drugs are being replaced.When explaining a drug to a patient:

- Introduce yourself.
- Check understanding about drugs and expectations (see *Explaining diseases*, p. 107).
- Check for allergies and contraindications.
- Explain what the drug is and its class.
- Explain the mechanism of action (MoA). How does the drug work? Use layman's terms, e.g. *it stops acid, opens airways, prevents your sugar levels from becoming too high.*
- Explain the **drug regime**:
  - How it is taken, e.g. swallowed, injected, etc.?
  - Does the patient need any special devices? If yes, see *Explaining devices*, p. 171.
  - How many times a day should it be taken?
  - When in the day should they be taking it?
  - Before or after food?
  - Should they avoid any over-the-counter medicines?
  - Should they avoid any foods, e.g. grapefruit with simvastatin?
  - Duration of the course of treatment.
- Explain any **side effects** of the drugs.
- Let the patient know if there is any **follow-up**, e.g. future blood tests to check levels, INR for warfarin.

- Explain if the medication interacts with other medication, e.g. interaction with the oral contraceptive pill or liver enzyme inducers/retardants.
- Consider **patient behaviour**: Is there anything the patient cannot do, for example, drinking alcohol whilst taking metronidazole?
- Inform the patient if there are any **lifestyle changes** that can be made in addition to the medication, for example, giving up smoking.
- Consent the patient to check that they are happy to proceed with the suggested treatment.
- Summarise, check understanding and remind them that the drug information leaflet will give useful information.
- Answer any questions and encourage patient involvement in medicine management.

EXPLAINING ATENOLOL

When explaining the drug atenolol:

- Introduce yourself.
- Check understanding about prescription and expectations. You may need to explain angina (see *Explaining angina*, p. 114).
- Check for any allergies and any contraindications (asthma, peripheral vascular disease, etc.).

Introduction

We are going to be prescribing you atenolol. This drug belongs to a class of drug called beta-blockers.

Mechanism of action

The drug works by stopping the heart beating fast, so reducing the energy needed to work. It therefore has a dual purpose in treating angina and lowering blood pressure.

Drug regime

- *Atenolol comes in tablet form – 25/50/100 mg dose tablets.*
- *Depending on the dosage regime, you normally take one or two tablets in the morning, with water. You may be asked to take two tablets 12 hours apart instead of the full amount in one go, although this is uncommon.*
- *Atenolol should be taken every day, with water, until the doctor stops it.*
- *It should not be stopped suddenly – it needs to be discontinued gradually.*

Side effects

People commonly complain of wheeziness, tiredness, cold peripheries and impotence; however, these side effects are generally tolerable. There should be some caution with the use of the drug in diabetic patients.

Drug interactions

Generally atenolol does not interact with other drugs or alcohol. Note – high risk of arrhythmias if given with diltiazem/verapamil.

Lifestyle

Changes can be implemented as well; the patient should be encouraged to take regular exercise for at least 30 minutes a day, stop smoking (talk about various smoking cessation programmes on offer), only drink alcohol in moderation, and cut down on the fat in their diet, as well as trying to eat healthily overall.

At the end of the interview

Summarise, check understanding and remind the patient that the drug information leaflet will give useful information.

Answer any questions the patient may have. Encourage patient involvement in medicine management. Remind the patient to request repeat prescriptions from the GP, giving sufficient notice.

EXPLAINING STATIN THERAPY

When explaining statin therapy to a patient:

- Introduce yourself.
- Give a brief summary about why you are prescribing it – *Your latest blood results showed that there was too much cholesterol in your blood. This is a risk factor for heart disease, stroke and heart attack. It is normal to prescribe a statin drug to patients with too much cholesterol, to help reduce their cholesterol level.*
- Check any allergies and contraindications.

Introduction

We are going to prescribe you atorvastatin/simvastatin, etc., *which is from a group of drugs called statins.*

Mechanism of action

This drug has been shown to be very effective in lowering the cholesterol level. It works by inhibiting the manufacturing of cholesterol within the body.

Drug regime

- *It is taken in tablet form in a variety of doses (simvastatin: 10/20/40/80 mg, atorvastatin 10/20/40 mg).*
- *It is normally taken, with water, at night before you go to bed.*
- *It is to be taken for the rest of your life, unless you are instructed by your doctor to stop.*

Side effects

There are very few side effects. However, you should be aware of two rare but serious ones, which affect the liver and muscles. If at any point, you take on a yellow tinge (become jaundiced) or start to notice muscular aches or wasting, it is important to stop the medication and inform your doctors as soon as possible.

Follow-up

Because of the side effects, you will need blood tests every 3 months, to test liver function and muscle enzyme activity. The blood tests are generally taken when you have been fasting for 12 hours.

Interactions

Generally, no interactions with other drugs are seen (avoid omeprazole), *and the drug is a good addition to any heart therapy regime.*

Lifestyle

Because this drug is part of a therapy to reduce the risk of heart disease, lifestyle changes should be implemented to reduce risk:

- *Exercise for 30 minutes a day (to raise a sweat).*
- *If you smoke, stop smoking.*
- *Only drink alcohol in moderation (21 units for women, 28 units for men per week: a pint of beer is 2 units; a glass of wine is 2 units).*
- *Follow a low-fat, low-salt diet (avoid adding salt to food).*
- *Lose weight and build fitness.*

At the end of the interview

Summarise, check understanding and remind the patient that the drug information leaflet will give useful information.

Ask – *Do you have any questions? We would like you to be involved in the management of your medicines.*

EXPLAINING SSRI DRUGS

When explaining an SSRI drug such as fluoxetine to a patient:

- Introduce yourself.
- Give a brief summary of why you are prescribing it – *I think, from what you told me, that you are suffering from depression. First line treatments, such as psychological therapy, have not helped yet. A drug called fluoxetine has been shown to be really useful in treating depression.*
- Check for any allergies and contraindications.

Introduction

Fluoxetine is a drug that helps fight depression. It belongs to a group called selective serotonin reuptake inhibitors (SSRIs).

Mechanism of action

Depression is thought to be caused by reduced levels of certain brain chemicals, such as serotonin and noradrenaline, in certain areas of the brain (see Explaining depression, *p. 111). Fluoxetine has been shown to restore a balance of these brain chemicals and so improve a patient's mood. Normally it takes up to 6 weeks for the drug to work and you must keep taking the drug during this time, even if you think it is not working.*

Drug regime

- *It is taken as a capsule, once a day, normally in the morning, with water.*
- *Doses are 20 mg and 60 mg.*

- *A syrup formulation is available for those unable to take capsules.*
- *You should not suddenly stop taking the medication, because there is a risk of withdrawal symptoms, characterised by sweating, anxiety and headaches.*

Side effects

One of the great benefits of the drug is that patients often say they find the side effects minimal, or at least tolerable. It has been reported that after starting the drug a few patients suffer from more suicidal thoughts and intentions and may think that their depression is worsening. This is not the case – it is the body redressing the imbalance of chemicals. If it is particularly bad, you should admit yourself to hospital for observation.

When patients are stable on the drug, common complaints are feeling sick, abdominal pain and discomfort, and a reduced appetite. The appetite effect is helpful for patients who want to lose weight as well.

It is important to mention the sexual side effects: people taking this drug often lose their libido or have decreased enjoyment of the sexual experience and orgasm, and this can be a common cause for stopping. But do not forget that lack of libido can be a symptom of depression anyway.

A rare but serious side effect, called serotonin syndrome, is caused by excessive serotonin in the brain, and if you develop this you will have to be admitted to hospital for monitoring and treatment.

In older patients, there may be a sodium imbalance, which may lead to dizziness, tiredness and confusion.

Follow-up

You do not need any more blood tests, but an occasional kidney function test will be useful. Your GP will monitor the progress of the depression. He may use a standard questionnaire to assess progress.

Different drugs within the same group work differently with different people – you may get on better with another drug if this one isn't helpful.

Interactions

There are very few interactions with other drugs. However, SSRIs are known to interact with some other psychiatric drugs, such as monoamine-oxidase inhibitors.

Other

To help treat depression, psychotherapy may help you to improve your outlook on life and yourself. Regular exercise can help, as can changing social circles, moving jobs or taking up new hobbies. Sometimes there is a need for consideration of major personal decisions, such as divorce. If appropriate, you can suggest bereavement counselling and self-help groups.

At the end of the interview

Summarise, check understanding and remind the patient that the drug information leaflet will give useful information.

Offer to answer any questions, and reassure the patient if doubts are expressed.

EXPLAINING ASTHMA MEDICATION

When explaining asthma medication to a patient:
- Introduce yourself.
- Give a brief summary of why you are prescribing it – *From what you've told me, I think that you are suffering from asthma. I think that two types of inhaler would be a good treatment.*
- Check any allergies and any contraindications.

Introduction

You will be prescribed two types of drug: salbutamol (Ventolin) and beclometasone (Qvar). Salbutamol belongs to a group of drugs called β_2-agonists. It is sometimes known as the reliever inhaler. Beclometasone is the preventer medicine and it is an inhaled steroid. Although it is a steroid, it does not have the same problems associated with steroid tablets when used long term.

Mechanism of action

The salbutamol works by affecting the β_2-protein in the airways, causing them to open up immediately, and bringing instant relief. The beclometasone works by taming the chemical processes that cause inflammation in the airways, preventing the airways from being easily stimulated and inflamed.

Drug regime

- *Both of these drugs are inhaled using special metered-dose inhalers (see Explaining inhalers, p. 177).*
- *Typically, the salbutamol comes in a light blue inhaler and the steroid comes in a brown inhaler.*
- *The salbutamol and the steroid drug can be taken up to a maximum of four times a day, and you take two puffs each time. You can take both these medications at the same time, but it is better to use the salbutamol 5 minutes before the beclometasone.*
- *The salbutamol can be taken if you have an asthma attack. You can also take two puffs if you feel wheezy between the scheduled doses. If you are having fewer attacks, you can cut down.*
- *A typical regime would be: one dose in the morning, one at lunch, one in the evening and one before you go to bed. However, you'll be directed by your asthma doctor.*

Side effects

People who take salbutamol can find it makes their heart beat faster and they may develop slight tremors. You may feel more anxious as well. This is more common when higher doses are used. Salbutamol can also reduce the amount of potassium in the blood, though this is only rarely a problem.

The steroid can cause a local infection in the throat, so you should gargle after inhaling. It must be stressed that short-term use of the inhaled steroid has been shown to have no long-term side effects. However, long-term use of inhaled steroids has been shown to have similar side effects to tablets (see section on oral steroids for side effects).

Using an inhaler spacer can reduce the amount of steroid left in the throat. Unfortunately, in the long term, inhaled steroids have been shown to have similar effects as oral steroids on bone and other body systems.

Follow-up

Generally, no follow-up is needed to monitor the effects of the medications themselves. Your GP will follow your asthma progress and decide if the drugs can be stopped or tailed off. They may monitor your asthma with a machine called a spirometer. You can also use a peak flow meter to monitor your treatment yourself.

Interactions

These drugs are generally safe with other drugs.

Lifestyle

To help combat asthma:
- *If you smoke, you should stop.*
- *Try to avoid triggers.*
- *Try to reduce dust levels using a damp duster, or vacuuming mattresses to reduce dust mite levels.*

At the end of the interview

- Summarise, check understanding and remind the patient that the drug information leaflet will give useful information.
- Answer any questions.

EXPLAINING ASPIRIN

When explaining aspirin to a patient:

- Introduce yourself.
- Give a brief summary of why you are prescribing it – *I think you are suffering from* (relevant disease) *and that aspirin would be a good treatment.*
- Check for any allergies and contraindications such as asthma, renal failure or gastrointestinal bleeding from ulcers.

Introduction

Aspirin is a well-established drug, which has been shown to have two effects: firstly it was found to be a pain killer and to reduce temperature, but then it was also found to thin the blood and has been very effective in lowering the risk of heart attacks and strokes.

Mechanism of action

Aspirin blocks a key protein that makes blood clotting factors and it reduces temperature. It is also known as salicylic acid.

Drug regime

- *A pill swallowed with food (breakfast, usually) after dissolving in water, one dose a day, taken in the morning.*
- *Aspirin comes in doses of 75 mg (one tablet) and one tablet is enough for heart disease protection. If it is used for fever control, then 300 mg is more usual.*

- It should not be taken **before** food (it irritates the lining of the stomach).
- As this drug is for your heart, it should be taken for life.

Side effects

Common side effects include nausea and vomiting. If you start vomiting blood or have strong indigestion-like pains, stop the aspirin and come to the hospital or seek advice from your GP as soon as possible. It's possible that the aspirin is irritating the lining of the stomach. That is why it is important to eat food before taking the tablet. Aspirin can also cause headaches and it can cause the airways in the lungs to narrow. Aspirin allergy is well recognised, compared to other drug allergies.

Follow-up

We will need to check your kidney function occasionally, but the main follow-up will be for your heart. You will need regular checks of your blood pressure, blood sugars and blood fats. There is a possibility that drugs to treat blood pressure and cholesterol will be added later.

Interactions

This drug's effects can be worsened if taken with other blood thinning drugs, the antidepressant citalopram, ibuprofen or diclofenac.

Lifestyle

Various lifestyle changes can be made to improve the prognosis of heart disease:

- Exercise for 30 minutes a day (to raise a sweat).
- If you smoke, stop smoking.

- *Only drink alcohol in moderation (21 units for women, 28 units for men per week: a pint of beer is 2 units; a glass of wine is 2 units).*
- *Follow a low-fat, low-salt diet (avoid adding salt to food).*

All of these will help you to lose weight and build fitness.

At the end of the interview

- Summarise, check understanding and remind the patient that the drug information leaflet will give useful information.
- Answer any questions.

EXPLAINING ORAL HYPOGLYCAEMICS (METFORMIN)

When explaining oral hypoglycaemics:

- Introduce yourself.
- Give a brief summary of why you are prescribing it – *Your recent results show that you suffer from type 2 diabetes and, in addition to controlling your diet, I would like you to try a drug called metformin to help control your sugar levels.*
- Check for any allergies and contraindications.

Introduction

We are going to introduce metformin into the management of your diabetes. It is a very widely used drug that helps reduce blood sugars further than diet control on its own. Unfortunately, with dietary control alone, your blood sugars are still quite high, so adding medication will help you to achieve better control.

Mechanism of action

Metformin works by reducing the production of sugar within the body from the breakdown of fats and proteins, and by making you more responsive to the insulin you already produce.

Drug regime

- *It is taken as a pill (500mg or 850mg) three times a day with water.*
- *It should be taken 20 minutes after food.*
- *You must take the medication at the right time, because it has a better effect on blood sugar if you do.*
- *It is best to gradually build up the dose over a few weeks.*
- *It may be used in conjunction with other medicines later.*

Side effects

The most common side effects are nausea and abdominal discomfort. It can cause quite severe diarrhoea, which may make it necessary for you to stop taking the drug. Diarrhoea generally settles with time. Metformin can also aid weight loss because it reduces appetite. Rarely, it can damage kidney function and, if that becomes the case, your medication will be changed.

Follow-up

It is essential to test your blood sugars regularly over the next month, with a home blood sugar kit, to see if this drug is helping. If it isn't, we can change drugs or add another one. Your GP or practice nurses will help monitor the diabetes. They will organise a special blood test called the glycosylated haemoglobin (HbA1c) test, which assesses the change in blood sugars over a 6-week period.

Interactions

Metformin does not generally interact with other drugs. This is useful in case you ever need to take cardiac drugs. It must not be used when there is already damage to the kidneys.

You should always tell a radiology department that you are on metformin because sometimes the dye used in some radiological tests can interact with the drug. A radiographer should always check whether you are on metformin.

Lifestyle

- *Follow a healthy, low-fat diet moderate in carbohydrates. Avoid fried fatty foods, chocolate, biscuits, crisps, etc.*
- *Your diet should contain a good amount of fruit and vegetables as well (five portions a day).*
- *Reduce the salt content of your diet.*
- *Take 30 minutes' moderately strenuous exercise each day.*
- *If you smoke, you should stop.*
- *Drink alcohol only in moderation (21 units for women, 28 units for men per week: a pint of beer is 2 units; a glass of wine is 2 units).*

All of these will aid loss of weight and build fitness.

At the end of the interview

- Summarise, check understanding, and remind them that the drug information leaflet will give useful information.
- Answer any questions and reassure the patient.

EXPLAINING THE COMBINED ORAL CONTRACEPTIVE PILL (OCP)

When explaining the oral contraceptive pill to a patient:

- Introduce yourself.
- Give a brief summary of why you are prescribing it – *You came today for contraceptive advice and from what you've told me, a good choice could be using the combined oral contraceptive pill.*
- Check any allergies and any contraindications (migraines/DVT).

Introduction

The oral contraceptive pill is 99% effective in preventing pregnancy when taken according to instructions and is the most common form of contraception used in the UK. However, it doesn't protect against sexually transmitted diseases.

Mechanism of action

The Pill works by suppressing the natural hormones that regulate the menstrual cycle, thus suppressing ovulation. Menstrual cycles become regular and uniform because of the cyclical dosing of the medication. The Pill has two hormones: oestrogen and progesterone.

Dose regime

The dose regime can be very complicated and should be fully understood before starting the medication:

- *You should take your pill once a day with water.*
- *The pattern is cyclical: 21 days of tablets and 7 days without. Some types of the Pill have seven dummy tablets so you would take a tablet every day.*
- *During the pill-free (or dummy pill) week you will have your menstrual bleed. The bleed is called a withdrawal bleed and is not due to ovulation.*
- *It is important to take the Pill at roughly the same time each day. With the Combined Pill you have until 12 hours after your normal time to take your pill, if you are to remain protected. For example, if you normally take it at 8 a.m. every day, you have until 8 p.m. to take it. We would encourage you to develop strategies to remember the time to take your pill at the same time each day.*
- *If you miss one or two doses then take your next pill as soon as you remember. You should use condoms for 7 days. If you miss three doses then it is best to seek advice from the GP, practice nurse or family planning clinic, and start again on a fresh packet. You should still use condoms. If you miss a pill at the end of the packet, you should carry on with the new packet, without the usual 7-day break. You will have no breakthrough bleed that month.*

Side effects

The Pill does not protect against sexually transmitted disease such as HIV. Women commonly complain of feeling sick when they first start taking the Pill. You may gain weight or notice a few more spots than usual. If you do vomit within 3 hours of taking one pill, then you need to follow the guidance for when you've missed one pill: use condoms for 7 days and take another tablet.

There are other possible severe side effects that you should be aware of:

- High blood pressure, which can lead to stroke or heart attack.
- Stickier blood, which can increase the risk of blood clots in the legs (DVT) and, more seriously, in the lungs.
  - **Emergency point**: If you have any pains in your calves, difficulty in breathing, coughing up blood or new chest pain, you must go to hospital immediately.
- Triggering the new onset of migraines.
- Development of breast lumps – in this case please seek advice from your GP.

Follow-up

Typically the GP will manage your contraception and, because there are many different types of Combined Pill, the amount of hormone in the Pill can be adjusted to reduce side effects.

Interactions

Like all other drugs, the Pill can interact with other drugs. For example, antibiotics can often reduce the effectiveness of the Pill. If you are taking antibiotics, you should use condoms for the amount of time you're taking them and up to 7 days afterwards.

If you are having planned surgery, you should stop the Pill around 4 weeks before the date of the surgery. If you have an episode of gastroenteritis, you must be aware that the absorption of the Pill *may be affected, you may get some spotting and you may need to take extra precautions.*

At the end of the interview

- Summarise, check understanding and remind the patient that the drug information leaflet will give useful information.
- Answer any questions.
- Remind patients to have a smear test regularly.

EXPLAINING WARFARIN

When explaining warfarin to a patient:

- Introduce yourself.
- Give a brief summary of why you are prescribing it – *We are giving you warfarin because you have a history of blood clots in your leg/lungs – because of your new valve – because of your irregular heart rhythm, etc.*
- Check any allergies and contraindications.

Introduction

Warfarin is a very effective drug for reducing blood clotting.

Mechanism of action

Warfarin works by blocking the production of key blood clotting factors, so that your blood runs more freely. In particular, it reduces vitamin K levels, so fewer clotting factors can be produced.

Dose regime

- *It is taken in the evening at around 6 p.m. and should be taken at the same time every day.*

- *It comes as a tablet and should be taken with water.*
- *The dose you take will be calculated during your visit to the anticoagulation clinic.*
- *Your dose is monitored by a special blood test called the INR.*
- *Tablets come in different colours and doses of 1 mg, 3 mg and 5 mg.*

Side effects

Because warfarin slows down clotting, you're more likely to bleed. People normally notice that they bruise more easily. More rarely, people suffer from rashes and allergic-type reactions to the drug. It can also have an unfavourable effect on fetuses. It can affect your liver (the organ where clotting factors are made).

Emergency point: If you start having nose bleeds, bleed from the mouth or back passage, or bruise very easily, you must go to the hospital immediately and seek guidance about stopping the warfarin. It could be that your blood is too thin. You will have your blood checked in hospital and a decision will be made there about the future dose. You should also go to hospital if your skin or eyes take on a yellow tinge (jaundice – a sign of liver damage).

Interactions

Because clotting factors are made in your liver, warfarin affects drugs that are broken down by the liver. This might affect other medications, so always advise your doctor and pharmacist that you are taking it. You should also avoid eating grapefruit.

Follow-up

Your blood clotting will need to be tested regularly, and this is done at special clinics in the hospital called anticoagulation clinics. They look at a measure of clotting called INR and give it a number range: typically your number should be between 2 and 3 or 3 and 4.

Based on your INR, the clinic will tell you the dosage of warfarin to be taken until the next test. The dose and the level are written in a yellow book called a warfarin book, which you should keep with you at all times.

Interactions

If you are planning on becoming pregnant, you should be aware that warfarin is known to have a strong effect on the fetus, so a lot of preplanning will need to be considered.

You should be wary of excessive physical activity because of the increased risk of injury and uncontrolled bleeding. This can be serious, especially in the case of head injuries.

At the end of the interview

- Summarise, check understanding and remind the patient that the drug information leaflet will give useful information.
- Answer any questions.

EXPLAINING STEROID USE

When explaining steroid use to a patient:

- Introduce yourself.
- Give a brief summary of why you are prescribing it.
- Check any allergies and contraindications.

Introduction

Steroids are used to reduce the inflammation of tissue. They can be used in addition to other drugs such as antibiotics in allergic infections or to reduce allergic skin problems.

Mechanism of action

Steroids are very effective at reducing the inflammation response of the body. However, because of the way the steroids work, the body will stop producing its own natural steroids if steroid drugs are used for long periods of time, and eventually the tablets will replace your own supply.

The following information is more advanced and may be suitable for a more informed patient – *The body produces its own steroids. This is controlled by the brain via a negative feedback process, i.e. when there are more steroids present in the body, it reduces steroid production. When additional steroids are given by tablets or injection, the body cannot differentiate between the artificial steroid and its own, and it will shut down its own natural steroid production.*

Drug regime

- You must take your steroids every day in the morning. This is to emulate the body's release of natural steroid, which is naturally highest in the early morning.
- Steroids come in tablet form and are swallowed with water, along with food. They are also available in soluble form.
- **Emergency point**: If you have been taking steroids for a long time, there is a high risk of developing a crisis if you forget to take your steroids. This is a medical emergency because your blood pressure drops and you have low blood sugar levels. It is potentially fatal.
- If it is decided that you don't need steroids any more, you must **not** stop them suddenly – a reducing regime is necessary, e.g. you will cut down by one pill per day at weekly intervals. It is important to wean yourself off the steroids slowly, particularly after being on them continuously for 3 months or more.

Side effects

There is an increased risk of infections, bruising and weight gain with higher doses of steroids. People sometimes comment that they change appearance, especially around the face. Another common problem is that steroids can thin the lining of the stomach, leading to severe indigestion and ulcers.

With long-term steroid use there is an increased risk of:
- fractures, due to bone thinning
- developing diabetes
- developing high blood pressure.

Additional regular drugs may be taken with the steroids, in order to protect the bones and reduce the risk of fractures. Regular medication to stop the risk of developing a stomach ulcer will also be given.

Follow-up

Because prescribed steroids are replacing the body's own supply, there is an extra need to get the dosage right. Your GP will monitor closely how your body is coping with the steroid and will also do regular checks on blood sugar and bones to monitor for side effects. You must tell your GP if you experience increased thirst or are passing urine more frequently. You must also tell your GP about the symptoms of any recurrent infections.

Lifestyle

- You should carry a **steroid card**, so that if you are taken into hospital it is immediately available to inform any further treatment decisions that may be affected by your steroids.
- You should also carry an **ampoule of steroid** with you at all times, in case one day you forget to take your normal dose and fall ill suddenly. You can crush the ampoule in your teeth to stop the crisis from developing.
- You must take twice your normal steroid dose when you have a fever.
- It is advisable to wear an SOS Talisman® identity locket. These are available commercially and may be worn around the neck or on a bracelet.

At the end of the interview

- Summarise, check understanding and remind the patient that the drug information leaflet will give useful information.
- Answer any questions.

Explaining device Z

EXPLAINING DEVICES

The principles of explaining devices are the same as *Explaining diseases*, p. 107, and *Explaining drugs*, p. 145.

The following template can be used for any device that may be presented to you:

- Introduce yourself to the patient.
- Check their understanding of the need for the device and their expectations.
- Show the patient the device and explain the key features.
- Find out about the patient's previous experience – *Have you ever seen one or do you know anyone who uses one?*
- Explain the **purpose** of the device, e.g. *to deliver medication/monitor treatment.*
- Slowly explain **how to use** the device, in a series of steps – *Firstly you insert the cartridge in here, then…*
- **Demonstrate** using the device: you may have a dummy device to use.
- Get the patient to use it in front of you in order to check their technique.
- Point out **common mistakes** made by patients and how to avoid them.
- Tell the patient about a suitable **regime** of using the device; e.g. blood pressure monitoring in the morning.
- Where they can obtain a device (e.g. prescription only for peak flow, health shops for blood pressure monitors).
- Consent the patient for use of the device.
- Give **general advice** regarding the condition (see *Explaining diseases*, p. 107) and the medication to be used in the device (see *Explaining drugs*, p. 145).
- Summarise briefly and answer any questions.

EXPLAINING GTN SPRAY

When explaining GTN spray to a patient:

- Introduce yourself.
- Check understanding for the spray and the patient's expectations.
- Show them the GTN spray and explain the key features; find out about previous experience.
- Explain: *The **purpose** of the spray is to deliver the medication glyceryl trinitrate (GTN), which opens up the vessels supplying the heart to relieve the angina pain.*

Explain how to use it

- *Give the bottle containing the medication a firm shake before you lift the cap.*
- *Open your mouth and lift your tongue onto the roof of your mouth.*
- *Then spray twice under your tongue.*
- *You'll notice the medication work within seconds and your chest pain will disappear.*
- *If the pain doesn't go after 15–30 seconds, then have another two sprays.*
- *Replace the cap after using the spray.*

Demonstrate using the spray and get the patient to use it in front of you to check their technique.

Advise the patient as follows:

- ***Most importantly**, if you notice that the spray does not help the angina even after three or four sprays, you should go to hospital straight away because there may be something more seriously wrong with your heart.*
- *After using the GTN spray, you might notice other effects such as your face warming up and being flushed, and you may have a minor headache. These side effects are only temporary and not a reason to stop using the spray. They usually disappear as*

you get used to the medicine. They are due to the local blood vessel opening in the whole of the head area.

- *If you are having continuing problems then you can contact our heart specialist nurse, or read the detailed pamphlet accompanying the spray.*

Common mistakes

The GTN spray is quite straightforward to use. However, the most common mistake people make is not spraying under the tongue. The medicine doesn't taste good and may make people retch.

Regime

You should use the spray when you experience the angina-like chest pain. If you notice you are using the spray more frequently, then you should see your doctor.

I will issue a prescription for the spray, and you can get repeat prescriptions from your GP once the bottle runs out.

General advice

- Explain angina (p. 114) and lifestyle changes to help combat ischaemic heart disease.
- Summarise briefly and answer any questions.

EXPLAINING INSULIN INJECTOR PENS

When explaining insulin injector pens to a patient:

- Introduce yourself.
- Check their understanding of the need for the pen and explain that the pen is needed to inject insulin to treat their diabetes (p. 125).
- Find out about their previous experience.
- Show them the insulin pen, and point out the key features – dial, needle, injecting mechanism – and explain how to use it.

It is very important to get the use of the pen right because of the need for lifelong use of insulin.

An injection regime will have been decided by the diabetes consultant. Check that you have the right pen and the correct type of insulin before demonstrating injection, as follows:

- *Adjust the counter on the pen to the number of units you should have for that time of the day.*
- *Inject the insulin in the fatty parts of the body; normally this is the fat part around the tummy area or the thighs.*
- *Grab hold of a good amount of fat and gently insert the needle part at right angles to the skin.*
- *Press the plunger down and the insulin will be injected in the body.*
- *Count to 10.*
- *Let go of the fatty part and remove the needle.*
- *Recap the insulin pen to prevent contamination.*

Demonstrate use of the pen on a dummy cushion or pad (don't prick yourself!). Get the patient to use it in front of you to check technique.

Common mistakes

- *Not changing the sites where the insulin injections are given. If you always use the same injection site, it will form scar tissue and harden, causing insulin lumps.*
- *Make sure you inject the correct number of units and the correct type of insulin at the appropriate time of the day for the best sugar control. If you use too high a dose of insulin, you risk your blood sugar being too low.*
- *Make sure that you don't withdraw the needle too soon; if you do, an incomplete insulin dose will be delivered.*
- *If you have difficulty mastering the technique, you should see the diabetes specialist nurse, who can go through the technique with you or try different pens.*

Regime

The diabetes consultant will have suggested a regime for the number of injections per day, how many units per injection and when you should take it. You should follow those instructions as closely as possible. You should also test your own blood sugars during the day before meals to see how effective your insulin regime is.

The insulin pens have to be prescribed; however, home testing blood sugar kits are available from pharmacists or we can issue you with one. The test strips for the machine are available on prescription.

General advice

- Give general advice regarding diabetes management.
- Summarise briefly and answer any questions.

EXPLAINING PEAK FLOW METERS

- Introduce yourself to the patient.
- Check their understanding of the meter and any expectations they may have.
- Show the patient the peak flow meter and point out the key features (mouthpiece/dial).
- Find out if they have any previous experience of the meters.
- Explain the **purpose** of the peak flow meter: to monitor their asthma condition and check on the effectiveness of any medication they may be taking.

Explain how to use the peak flow meter

Demonstrate the use of the peak flow meter:

- *Attach the mouthpiece into the main body (if unattached).*
- *Set the dial to zero and hold the meter without obstructing the dial.*

- *Stand up and then take deep breaths to clear your lungs.*
- *Take a deep breath in and hold it.*
- *Place the mouthpiece in your mouth and form a tight seal around it.*
- *Blow out as **hard and fast** as you can, without impeding the dial.*
- *Make a note of the number and then repeat twice more to get three readings.*
- *Your best reading is the one you should note down in a peak flow diary.*
- *A nose clip can be used if you find you breathe out through the nose.*

Get the patient to use it in front of you to check technique.

Common mistakes

- Coughing or not breathing out as hard as they can.
- Breathing in (!) when they should be breathing out.
- Not setting the dial to zero; many people forget about this.
- Placing their fingers in the tract of the dial and thereby obstructing it.

Problems can be addressed by reading the information accompanying the meter or by consulting the specialist asthma nurse.

Regime

*You should use this device twice a day – once in the morning and once in the evening – especially after a change in a medication. You do **not** have to use it every day; three times a week is adequate. You should make a note of the values in a diary and show them to your GP/consultant at your next visit.*

Normally you can get a peak flow on prescription; however you can also buy them at health shops.

General advice

- Give general advice regarding asthma.
- Summarise briefly and answer any questions.

EXPLAINING INHALERS

There are many different types of inhaler, but they can be broadly split into two categories: inhalers where you have to dispense the medication while using them (metered dose inhalers) and inhalers that have a breath-activated trigger. The metered dose inhaler is the more common of the two.

When explaining a metered dose inhaler to a patient:

- Introduce yourself to the patient.
- Check their understanding of the need for the device.
- Show them the inhaler, pointing out the important parts (mouthpiece and medication cartridge).
- Find out about the patient's previous experience of inhalers.
- Explain the **purpose** of the inhaler – *it administers asthma drugs by allowing you to inhale them directly into your lungs.*
- *Inhalers represent different types of medication: the blue ones are the relievers and the others, such as the brown ones, are the preventers.*

Explain how to use the inhaler

- *If the cartridge has fallen out of the dispenser, re-attach it and press down twice to ensure a good connection.*
- *Stand up or sit up straight and breathe in and out deeply.*
- *Place your mouth round the mouthpiece, forming a tight seal around it.*

- *While you breathe in, press down the dispenser/canister so that you inhale the medication as you breathe and it goes deep into your lungs.*
- *Hold your breath for 10 seconds after breathing in, so that the medication can settle in the lungs.*
- *Breathe out slowly through your nose.*
- *Repeat if a second puff is needed.*
- *After using the brown inhaler (an inhaled steroid), you should gargle with water.*

When you have demonstrated its use, get the patient to use it in front of you to check their technique.

Common mistakes

- *Not coordinating breathing in and pressing the cartridge down; this can lead to the medication being left in your mouth.*
- *Breathing out too soon will reduce the amount of the drug in the lungs.*
- *Not gargling with water after taking the steroid can lead to throat infections.*
- *If you're having difficulties, especially with coordinating pressing the cartridge and breathing, then you can try another type of inhaler.*

Regime

The number of times you should take the drug is determined by your prescription. It may vary from once in the morning to up to four times a day.

Since this is a device to deliver medication, it is only available via prescription.

General advice

Give general advice regarding asthma (p. 108) and asthma medication (p. 152).

Summarise briefly and answer any questions they may have.

Explaining a spacer

This is a common device, often used in conjunction with an inhaler. The object of the spacer is to remove the need for pressing down on the canister while inhaling. It has also been shown to lower the risk of throat infections.

The spacer is designed with a one-way valve where the patient inhales and, at the other end, an entry hole for the inhaler. The patient sets up the equipment first and then places the inhaler in the entry point. With their mouth over the inhalation point, they spray the inhaler so that the drug enters the large chamber. They should then breathe in and out slowly four or five times so that all of the drug is inhaled.

EXPLAINING ADRENALINE PENS

When explaining adrenaline pens to a patient:
- Introduce yourself to the patient.
- Check the patient's understanding of their need for the adrenaline pen.
- Show them a pen, pointing out the key features (needle/ release button).
- Find out if they have any previous experience of adrenaline pens.
- Explain the purpose of the pen – *The pen is designed to deliver adrenaline and is used if you develop an acute allergic reaction. The adrenaline will temporarily stop your blood pressure dropping, which will support your heart and brain. After using the pen you should go straight to the hospital emergency department for further treatment. If necessary, an ambulance should be called.*

Explain the use of the pen

- *The technique for using the pen is very easy and it can save your life.*
- *When you start experiencing the symptoms of allergy (chest tightening, difficulty breathing, sudden and strong itchiness, swelling of the skin, etc.) you should use the pen. There is a risk of sudden deterioration from these relatively minor symptoms to something more serious.*
- *Firstly call for help from nearby people or emergency services.*
- *Pull off the cap of the pen to expose the needle.*
- *Immediately stab the needle into the thigh area.*
- *Press the plunger firmly until all the contents have been expelled.*
- *Remember that adrenaline can have side effects, which include palpitations and breathing problems.*

When you have demonstrated the use of the pen, get the patient to use it in front of you to check technique.

Common mistakes

There are very few potential mistakes. However, care must be taken to avoid the following:

- *Using expired adrenaline pens: you should check the best-before date regularly and replace the pen if necessary. Out of date adrenaline loses its potency.*
- *Injecting in the peripheries (hands or feet) where circulation isn't good. The adrenaline will cause peripheral blood vessels to constrict and potentially cause irreversible damage to the fingers or toes.*

Regime

There is no strict regime; you should use it if you start experiencing the symptoms of being exposed to your allergen (shortness of breath, wheeze, feeling faint, palpitations, swelling of the tongue or face).

Adrenaline pens are typically dispensed at the pharmacy. You should carry one with you at all times. You can also wear a bracelet, which will inform third parties of your allergy and the allergen. Obtain a new prescription for a replacement pen when the expiry date is reached.

General advice

- Give general advice regarding anaphylaxis and allergic reactions.
- Summarise and answer any questions.

8

Explaining procedures

EXPLAINING PROCEDURES – GENERAL ISSUES

All procedures that are relatively complex, i.e. those that involve multiple stages such as sedation, intervention and recovery, will probably need to be explained by the person performing the procedure and have explicit consent forms signed. Earlier in the book we mentioned the basic principles for informed consent, p. 11. To refresh your memory these are:

- Introduce yourself.
- Check understanding and expectations.

Explain to the patient:

- the procedure and who will undertake it
- the **reasons** why this procedure is being carried out
- the **benefits** of the procedure
- the **risks** involved in the procedure
- the **methodology** of how the procedure/surgery will be performed:
  - duration of the procedure
  - preparation work, e.g. coming in 1 or 2 days before the procedure, prophylactic antibiotics
  - what the procedure will involve (logistics)
- **follow-up** advice after the procedure and management afterwards
- what will happen if the patient chooses not to have the procedure
- **alternative possibilities** to the procedure being considered.

Summarise and answer any questions the patient may have.

Consent

Although we have concentrated on procedures that need a consent form, even for procedures as simple as venepuncture, you should always gain verbal consent about the need for the procedure and:

- explain what you're doing as you're doing it
- give simple instructions – *Can you straighten your arm and make a fist? I'm going take blood from your elbow region.*
- give prior warning of pain or discomfort – *You will feel a little sharp scratch as I put the needle in your arm.*
- warn about possible side effects – *You might notice a little bruise where the needle went in, which should go in a couple of days.*

EXPLAINING LIGHT SEDATION

All of the following procedures require light sedation and some general advice should be given when a patient undergoes light sedation.
You should advise the patient:

- to rest for the remainder of the day
- not to drive for at least 24 hours
- to have someone accompany them home and to check up on them for at least 24 hours after a procedure
- to avoid any alcohol and illicit drugs
- not to work with heavy machinery or technically demanding/dangerous tasks until the effect of the sedation has worn off.

EXPLAINING CENTRAL LINE PLACEMENT

Introduction

This is a procedure that can be done on a ward or in a surgical theatre setting. For this example we will assume it will take place in theatre:

- Introduce yourself.
- Check understanding and expectations.
- Explain – *The procedure is to place a central line into your neck vein and it will be done by an experienced operator, such as a registrar.*

Reasons

The team has decided that we need to place a central line directly into your neck vein. A central line is very similar to the tubes you have in your arms.

The reasons why we want to put a line in the neck vein are that:

- *you don't have good veins in your arms to put in lines to give you fluid, blood and medication*
- *we may need to administer special drugs, e.g. chemotherapy, through this line; these would be toxic to the arm veins.*

Benefits

There are several advantages: the line can stay in for many days without being replaced. It reduces the risk of destroying the arm veins, and we can remove blood and put substances down the same line so there is no need to use needles to take blood. The line is quite easy to remove.

Risks

- *The common risks include: discomfort during the procedure, a risk of infection either at the time of insertion or later on (though a sterile technique is used) and a risk of bleeding.*
- *You'll have the line taped to your neck, which some people find irritating, and a little scar may ultimately be present later.*
- *More serious risks include a lung puncture during insertion of the line, due to the close proximity of the vein to the top of the*

lungs. If this should happen, it is easy to remedy; a chest drain may need to be inserted to allow the lung to re-inflate.

- The vein and artery lie next to each other and it's possible that we might go into the artery instead. This is very rare, but it should be mentioned. Should this happen, the line will be removed immediately and pressure will be applied so that the bleeding stops.
- There is a possibility that we may not be able to find a neck vein; if that's the case, the medical team will consider alternative options.

Methodology

- **Duration** – The procedure will take around 30 minutes to perform and be undertaken by an experienced operator.
- **Logistics** – We will be giving you some light sedation to help you relax. It will also help to relax the muscles in your neck.
- A sterile environment will be created before we insert the line.
- You will be lying down throughout and you will need to turn your head to expose the veins.
- Some local anaesthetic will be administered in the area to numb it before any needles are inserted.
- We will need to make a small cut in the skin in order to insert the line.
- Firstly, we insert a needle into the vein, which acts as a guide for the line.
- The line is then gradually inserted in the vein.
- The end of the line will be taped or sutured to your neck to prevent accidental dislodgement. It will remain there until it is no longer needed.

After the procedure

You will be taken for a chest X-ray after the procedure to check that the line was inserted correctly and to confirm its position. You will then remain in hospital to continue the rest of your treatment.

Alternatives

Without the line we could not give you the correct drugs for your condition or give you the necessary fluids to help you get better. There are no good alternatives that don't require specialist help from intensive care.

At the end of the interview

Summarise and answer any questions the patient may have. Offer them a procedure fact sheet.

EXPLAINING ANGIOGRAMS

When explaining angiograms to a patient:
- Introduce yourself.
- Check understanding and expectations.
- Explain – *We would like to perform an angiogram. The procedure will be undertaken by a consultant cardiologist.*

Reasons

You were admitted for chest pain, which the doctors thought could be due to your angina (heart muscle cramp). Tests have indicated an abnormality to the blood vessels of the heart.

Benefits

An angiogram allows the doctor to observe the circulation in the heart blood vessels, see any blockages and assess how severe your heart disease is. It will act as a reference point for any future tests.

Should the doctor performing the procedure decide, they can put in stents to open up the blood vessels or use a balloon to increase their diameter (angioplasty). Stents are small tube-like objects, which allow blood to flow and keep the artery open.

Risks

The risks include pain, infection, swelling and scarring at the entry site of the wire. In rare cases the wire passing through can aggravate a current circulation obstruction and precipitate a heart attack. Because the wire and probe enter the heart vessels, it is possible to damage the blood vessels.

Stents have been known to trigger heart attacks. The dye used can have side effects, such as hot flushes, and can interact with some diabetic medication. The dye can contain iodine and elements of seafood; patients with allergies to these should tell the doctor.

Methodology

Duration

This procedure generally takes a whole day; this includes any transport to a specialist site, preparation for the local sedative, the procedure and recovery. The operator is going to be a senior heart specialist, such as a cardiac registrar or consultant. There is of course a back-up team present should anything go wrong. It is very rare for things to go wrong.

Preparatory work

A week before the test, you will be asked to have some blood tests. The results of these will determine if this test can proceed. You should stop your blood-thinning medication a few days before the procedure (e.g. warfarin). You should stop eating at least 8 hours before the test.

Logistics

You will be fully monitored throughout the whole procedure. Local anaesthetic is applied to the inner thigh and a needle is passed into a main artery of the leg. A wire with a special probe is passed up through the artery and aimed towards the heart. Some dye is injected and X-ray pictures (with a camera in theatre) will be taken to allow full visualisation of the coronary arteries. The dye can cause hot flushes in some patients.

Should the operator decide, they can place stents to allow the arteries to be widened or may manually try to widen them by inflating a balloon.

After the procedure

You will be closely monitored during your recovery, then sent back to the ward. A doctor will assess you and your wound site before you go home.

Follow-up

After the test, a heart specialist will analyse the images. You will be followed up by a heart specialist, who will also monitor any worsening of your symptoms. If results show only minor disease or even no disease, then your GP will continue to manage your angina. If stents are put in, then you may be given extra medication to prevent clots forming around the stents and triggering a heart attack.

Alternatives

If doctors do not do an angiogram, then they will not know if your symptoms originate from your heart and will not be able to properly assess how severe the disease is. There are no alternatives to looking directly at the arteries of the heart. The most definitive treatment would be heart surgery; however, this carries considerable risk.

At the end of the interview

Summarise and answer any questions the patient may have. Offer them a procedure fact sheet.

EXPLAINING EXERCISE STRESS TESTS (EST)

When explaining the exercise stress test to a patient:

- Introduce yourself.
- Check the patient's prior knowledge and expectations.
- Explain – *The procedure is an exercise stress test, which will be performed by an experienced operator.*

Reasons

The EST is an investigation used to look at your heart during physical stress. The reason for doing it is that by looking at the heart we can spot any irregular rhythms that arise when you exercise. We can then grade your angina and monitor your progress after a heart attack.

Benefits

We can directly scan the heart during physical stress, look for any abnormalities that might appear when the heart is deprived of oxygen and see where specifically in the heart they appear. We can also look at the condition of the heart after your heart attack.

Risks

There are some risks:

- *Commonly, you'll feel tired and a bit short of breath; you might retch and your muscles and joints might ache afterwards. This is very common after the exercise.*
- *Rarely, but seriously, a heart attack may occur; you'll get sudden chest pain and have difficulty breathing.*
- *Irregular rhythms in the heart.*
- *Very rarely, death or long-term damage from a heart attack or irregular heartbeat.*

Methodology

Duration

The test will take roughly a couple of hours to allow for monitoring before and after exercise.

Preparatory work

No special measures need to be taken before the day; however, it is advisable to wear loose clothing and good footwear.

Logistics

- *The EST will be done by a trained technician, who is experienced and knows what to do in an emergency. If need be, we can call upon additional doctors for assistance in an emergency.*
- *Various electrodes will be connected to your chest: these take electrical readings of your heart (ECG).*
- *Before you start you will have a baseline ECG and blood pressure readings.*
- *You will then step onto a treadmill, where you will have to start walking against some resistance. The test programme gradually increases the speed and incline, thereby increasing the amount of effort you have to make. Eventually you might be running.*
- *Throughout the exercise you will have your blood pressure monitored and ECGs done. The overall situation is monitored by the technician.*
- *If you experience chest pain, become very short of breath, or feel wheezy, faint or about to pass out, then you must tell the technician, who will stop the test. They will also stop the test if they notice irregularities in your blood pressure or heart rhythm.*

After the procedure

You will continue to have regular monitoring of blood pressure and ECGs for around 20 minutes afterwards. The test will be interpreted and the results sent to your doctor.

Alternatives

If we didn't do the procedure, then we would not be able to formally diagnose any problems with your heart. This would delay appropriate treatments.

Should the exercise test not be possible, then we can administer drugs to stress the heart and monitor it. We can also do an ultrasound to assess the function of heart. However, the results are most telling when the heart undergoes real exercise stress.

At the end of the interview

Summarise and answer any questions the patient may have. Offer them a procedure fact sheet.

All of the following procedures require light sedation and it needs to be remembered that there is additional general advice to be given.

EXPLAINING OESOPHAGOGASTRODUODENOSCOPY (OGD) FOR EPIGASTRIC PAIN

When explaining oesophagogastroduodenoscopy (OGD) for gastric pain to a patient:

• Introduce yourself.
• Check the patient's prior knowledge and expectations.

Procedure

The test you are having is a camera test called oesophagogastroduodenoscopy (OGD for short) and it will be performed by an experienced surgeon/gastroenterologist with support from the nursing staff.

Reasons

You need this test because:

- *you are experiencing bleeding*
- *you may have ulcers*
- *you need to have the end opening of the stomach opened up*
- *you need a stent to be placed in the gullet to allow food to pass.*

We want to be able to look directly at your gullet, stomach and intestine. No other test allows us to do this.

Benefits

The camera allows the operator to:

- *look directly at the sites*
- *take samples when needed, at various sites*
- *perform any necessary corrective measures, such as placing stents to open up the gullet or cauterising the bleeding areas etc.*

Risks

One common complaint is that people may gag on the tube during the procedure. This is managed by using some anaesthetic spray at the back of the throat. However, the spray can lead to decreased sensation of swallowing. You may also experience a sore throat after OGD because a tube has been passed through your throat.

Because air is often pumped in during the procedure, you may feel bloated and may experience increased belching. This is very common and will pass quickly.

Rarely, the oesophagus and the bowel can be narrowed and there may be some mild bleeding as the tube passes through. Very rarely, the tube may perforate the oesophagus. Equally rarely, the tube may go into the lungs instead of the oesophagus, because they are very close together at the back of the throat. If this happens, the tube is immediately pulled out and the insertion procedure started again, but it may lead to an increased risk of a chest infection. In rare cases, patients may develop an allergic reaction to the sedative used to relax them.

Methodology

Duration

You should come in on the day of the procedure. The procedure will take around 1 hour, but you will need to take the whole day off to allow for waiting and recovery.

Preparatory work

You should not eat or drink for around 8 hours before the procedure. If the procedure is scheduled in the morning, eat nothing from midnight. If it is scheduled in the afternoon, you can have a light breakfast, but nothing from then on.

Logistics

You will be given some light sedation, which will help you relax. You will be placed on your left side and some local anaesthetic will be sprayed onto the back of your mouth to numb it. A small tube with a diameter of a penny coin will be placed into your mouth and when it hits the back of the throat, you'll be asked to swallow in order to get it into your gullet. The tube will be passed down into your stomach, and your stomach may be inflated with air to allow better views. Depending on how well you tolerate the tube, it may be further advanced into your intestines. The operator may decide to take photographs of the inside and may take some samples of tissues and carry out other procedures.

After the procedure

You will be placed in a recovery room for a few hours for the sedation to wear off. You will feel bloated and may well burp and pass wind. The doctor will analyse the results of the test and send them back to your consultant/GP, who will arrange further appointments.

Give further advice to the patient on recovery from the light sedation (see p. 186).

Alternatives

Other tests that can be performed are barium dye tests and CT scans. However, these tests do not allow direct visualisation or the ability to take samples. The most definitive procedure is surgery; however, this carries considerable risk.

At the end of the interview

Summarise and answer any questions the patient may have. Offer them a procedure fact sheet.

EXPLAINING COLONOSCOPY/FLEXI-SIGMOIDOSCOPY (C/FS) FOR PR BLEEDING

When explaining C/FS to a patient:

• Introduce yourself.
• Check prior knowledge and expectations.

Note that there is a possible diagnosis of bowel cancer with this test, so this may be a delicate situation.

Procedure

The test you are having is a camera test called colonoscopy and flexi-sigmoidoscopy: a C and FS. It will be performed by an experienced specialist with support staff.

Reasons

We need to do this procedure to investigate the bleeding from your back passage/need to investigate the mass seen on the CT scan and take samples. Colonoscopy will allow us to view right round the large bowel. Flexi-sigmoidoscopy will allow us to see the rectum and about 1 metre upwards from there.

Benefits

C/FS will allow us to look directly inside the bowel and colon. We can take photographs for further analysis or take samples of tissues for analysis, if needed.

Risks

The main problems are:
- *It is an uncomfortable procedure, though not painful.*
- *Commonly, patients pass wind and get crampy pain, since air is pumped into the bowel to give a better view. You may also get bleeding from the anus and in your stool, because of trauma from friction between the bowel and the tube.*
- *Infection can arise due to the introduction of an object into your body.*
- *Because we are inserting a tube into the bowel, there is a very small risk that we could go through the bowel wall and cause a perforation. This is rare, but could require emergency surgery if it happened. If you have profuse bleeding from the anus, or develop a high temperature, you should consult a doctor.*
- *Problems with the sedative may include including feeling sick and vomiting, or an allergic response.*

Methodology

Duration

The procedure will take up to an hour; however, time for waiting and recovery means the whole experience could take up to half a day.

Preparatory work

For flexi-sigmoidoscopy you will need bowel preparation to clear out the bowel, which can be done with enemas or tablets placed inside the anus to stimulate defecation.

For colonoscopy, before you come in, you will need to take laxatives to clear your bowel out. The laxatives are taken over 24 hours. They can be quite strong and may disturb your daily bowel routine. It is important to drink plenty of water to prevent dehydration. You will not be allowed to eat from midnight before the procedure, but you will be allowed sips of water.

Logistics

Before the procedure, you will be given a sedative to help you relax. It will be an uncomfortable, but not painful, procedure. You will be lying on your left-hand side, with your knees into your chest. A narrow tube will be placed into the bowel; it allows visual images of the gut lining to be seen by the operator. The operator will push the tube into the bowel and will have to manipulate it according to your individual anatomy. He may blow in air at the same time to clear the view and may also squirt water into the bowel passage.

The operator may take photographs and samples of tissue for further analysis. If there is any bleeding, we can cauterise the area with a laser to stop it. If it's very painful, you can tell the operator and they will stop.

After the procedure

You will be placed in recovery for a few hours waiting for the sedative to wear off. (Give further information about light sedation, see p. 186.)

The samples and photos will be analysed, and your GP/consultant will contact you with a follow-up appointment to discuss results and further plans.

Alternatives

We can do dye tests and scans, but no other procedure offers the ability to see the bowel directly and take samples or photos of the area at the same time. The most definitive approach is with surgery, but this carries considerable risk.

At the end of the interview

Summarise and answer any questions the patient may have. Offer them a procedure fact sheet.

EXPLAINING BRONCHOSCOPY FOR HAEMOPTYSIS

When explaining bronchoscopy for haemoptysis:
- Introduce yourself.
- Check prior knowledge and expectations.
- Note that there is a possible diagnosis of lung malignancy with this test, so please proceed with caution.

Procedure

Explain that bronchoscopy is a camera technique to look directly in the airways and will be performed by an experienced operator, such as a chest physician, with support nursing staff. There are two types of bronchoscope: flexible and rigid. The flexible version is most commonly used now.

Reasons

We need to be able to look at the lungs using a special camera called an endoscope. We can look at lung tissue directly and take samples of any lesion and surrounding lung tissues.

Stents can also be put in to keep airways open, should that be necessary.

Benefits

This procedure allows the operator to directly visualise lung tissue and to take samples and photos of the airways. It is generally a safe procedure and it is widely used.

Risks

It is very common to have a sore throat due to the irritation from the bronchoscopy tube. Other common risks include possible bleeding, especially if samples are taken. Also, the tube may introduce infection to the lungs.

Rarely, perforation of the lung tissue can occur. There is also a chance that the lung may collapse after the procedure, but that is rare.

You may also have a reaction to the sprays and sedative.

Methodology

Duration

The procedure may only take 30 minutes. However, time is spent waiting and in recovery and you should allow half a day in all.

Preparatory work

Please do not eat or drink anything for around 8 hours before the procedure. If the procedure is in the morning, eat nothing from midnight. If your procedure is scheduled for the afternoon, you can take a light breakfast in the morning.

Logistics

You will be lying down for the procedure. You will be given some medication to reduce the saliva in your mouth and a sedative to help you relax. You will also have a spray, which will numb the back of your mouth and nostrils. A narrow tube will be passed through your nostril and down into your windpipe towards to the lungs.

A camera within the tube can take pictures. The operator can see the lung tissue, take samples, place stents and take photographs. When we take samples, bleeding can occur, although it will be minor.

Your breathing will be monitored throughout and you will be given extra oxygen; however there should be minimal disturbance to your ability to breathe.

After the procedure

You will be in recovery for a few hours, waiting for the sedative to wear off. Gradually, swallowing and breathing should become easier. Because of the trauma to your windpipe and any samples we take, you will probably cough and you might bring up some phlegm with blood in it. You may also have a sore throat for a few days.

Include any advice on light sedation (see p. 186).

You should come back to the hospital if you suffer from a new fever, or if you are vomiting large amounts of blood or having new difficulty in breathing.

Follow-up

Your results will be analysed and your consultant will arrange a follow-up appointment to discuss the findings and further treatment options. The samples will be sent to a laboratory for analysis.

Alternatives

If we didn't do this test, then we would not be able to take samples or see the type or extent of the lump. There is an alternative to the procedure, called fine-needle aspiration, in which we scan the lungs and use a fine needle to suck out a small sample. However, the disadvantages of that procedure are that we can't see if the lump is attached to any other structures, and it may not be feasible to reach the lump.

At the end of the interview

Summarise and answer any questions the patient may have. Offer them a procedure fact sheet.

EXPLAINING ERCP FOR GALLSTONES

When explaining ERCP (endoscopic retrograde cholangio-pancreatography) for gallstones to a patient:
- Introduce yourself.
- Check understanding and expectations.

Procedure

The test you will be having is called an ERCP. It will be performed by an experienced operator such as a gastroenterologist/surgeon.

Reasons

We need to explore the ducts around your gall bladder. This will involve investigation of the pancreas as well. Some gallstones are small enough to pass out of the gall bladder, through the drainage system and into the bowel. However, sometimes the stones get caught in the ducts near the bowel and cause symptoms like yours. The ERCP will specifically explore this area and deal with any problems.

Benefits

We can look directly at the drainage ducts and will be able to take X-ray pictures. We can also use a balloon, which acts like a brush, to clear out the tube. We may decide to place a stent in a duct to keep it open and let any remaining stones and debris pass. Samples of tissue can also be taken, should the need arise. All of these techniques are possible with the ERCP. It is generally a very safe procedure and is widely used.

Risks

There are a few risks associated with the procedure:

- *There may be a reaction to the sedative used or to the dye used to take the picture.*
- *There is a medium risk that you could develop inflammation of the pancreas (again). If this happened, you would need to be kept in hospital.*
- *There may be some (minimal) internal bleeding.*
- *Because the camera has to pass through many structures to reach the duodenum, it can cause damage, although this rarely happens. In very rare cases, an operation may be needed to correct any damage.*
- *The operator may not be able to access the gall bladder ducts, due to a gallstone, or there may be so much debris in the tubes that it cannot be cleared out straight away by your body. This may lead to a return of your symptoms. With all foreign objects and trauma, there is a risk of infection.*

Methodology

Duration

ERCP will take around 2 hours to perform; however, you should allow time in recovery (1–2 hours) and waiting time. You will need to take a few days off work.

Preparatory work

You will need to come in the night before the ERCP. We do not allow you to eat or drink for 8–12 hours before the procedure. You will be given some preventative antibiotics before the procedure. You may have some blood taken to check your liver function and blood clotting ability.

If the procedure is in the afternoon, then a light breakfast can be eaten.

Logistics

- *ERCP is an uncomfortable procedure, but not painful.*
- *You will be taken to a unit and be given some light sedation to help you relax.*
- *You will also have a numbing spray applied to the back of your mouth. This should reduce the risk of you gagging.*
- *The operator will then pass a narrow tube past your gullet and stomach to the gall bladder region. The tube acts as a lens for the camera outside. The operator uses the camera pictures to guide them. They will also blow air to help guide the tube through.*
- *Within the tube, a smaller extension will come out and be inserted into the gall bladder ducts where the operator will inject a dye in order to be able to take an X-ray of the area.*
- *The operator may decide to insert a stent or use a balloon to clear out the drainage system.*
- *Afterwards, the operator will remove all the tubes.*

After the procedure

You will be permitted to rest in recovery to allow the sedation to wear off (see Explaining light sedation, p. 186). After the procedure, it is best that you take lots of fluid but no food. If at any time you have sudden abdominal pain, or start vomiting and feeling sick, please tell the staff immediately, as your symptoms could be due to pancreatic inflammation. If you start vomiting blood, you should see a doctor straight away. If you develop a new fever after you leave the hospital, you should return to the GP or hospital.

Follow-up

Once you are at home, your consultant will review the test findings and ask to see you in a follow-up clinic to discuss the results and further treatment.

Alternatives

There is no other test that allows us to see the area and treat it there and then. There are more detailed scans available, such as MRI, but they do not allow any correction to be done.

At the end of the interview

The doctor performing the procedure will see you on the day and explain in more detail what I've just told you. You will be asked to sign the consent form.

Summarise and answer any questions the patient may have. Offer them a procedure fact sheet.

EXPLAINING LUMBAR PUNCTURE

Lumbar puncture (LP) rarely needs an explicit consent form, but it is very complicated and is often a cause of concern for patients.

When explaining lumbar puncture to a patient:

- Introduce yourself.
- Check understanding before proceeding. Note that there is a potential diagnosis of multiple sclerosis with this test, so proceed with caution.
- Check if the patient has had a CT scan (there is a potential risk for cerebral herniation with increased intracranial pressure).

Procedure

We want to perform a procedure called a lumbar puncture, a technique to sample the fluid surrounding the brain and spinal cord.

Reasons

We would like to analyse the fluid because we think there could be an infection. We would also like to measure proteins and other markers of specific conditions within it.

Benefits

This is the only procedure whereby we can directly access the fluid for analysis and give a definite diagnosis. It does not last long and is not normally painful.

Risks

- *The procedure can occasionally be painful.*
- *There is a risk of infection, pain and local bleeding.*
- *Most commonly, patients may feel a tingling sensation in the legs because the needle is brushing against a nerve.*
- *Afterwards, some patients complain of a headache, which can be severe and last for several days. This can be relieved with simple painkillers.*
- *In rare cases, the needle can hit a major blood vessel or the spinal cord.*

Methodology

Duration

The procedure takes around 20 minutes for the doctor to do.

Preparatory work

No special requirements are needed and the procedure can be done at the bedside in sterile conditions.

Logistics

- *You will need to lie still on your left side with your knees held up into your chest.*
- *A sterile area will be created around the lower back.*
- *The clinician will give a local anaesthetic in the lower back to numb the area.*
- *The operator will proceed to insert a needle into your lower back and measure the pressure of the cerebrospinal fluid around your spine and brain.*
- *You will experience a lot of tugging and pulling in your lower back, which will be uncomfortable.*
- *If the procedure is very painful, and you notice strange sensations in your legs, please tell the operator immediately.*
- *The operator will remove around 5 ml of spinal fluid. This will be sent off to the laboratory for analysis.*
- *The operator will remove the needle, put further pressure on the entry site and put a plaster over it.*

After the procedure

You will need to lie on your back for a few hours and take plenty of fluids. You can also take simple painkillers. This will reduce the likelihood of headache.

If you notice that you cannot move your legs or if you have a persistent tingling sensation, please report this to the nurses as soon as possible.

Follow-up

Since this is almost certainly an inpatient test, the fluid samples will be sent for testing for proteins, sugar levels and infection. We will come back to you with the results. To avoid headache, or treat it if you do get one, you should remain lying flat and take some water and painkillers.

Alternatives

Lumbar puncture is the only way of directly examining the spinal fluid. Other scans and blood tests can only suggest a diagnosis. There are no alternatives.

At the end of the interview

The doctor performing the procedure will see you on the day, explain in more detail what I've just told you and ask you to sign a consent form.

Summarise and answer any questions the patient may have. Offer them a procedure fact sheet.

9 Explaining surgical operations

EXPLAINING SURGICAL OPERATIONS – GENERAL ISSUES

The approach to explaining surgical operations is almost identical to that for explaining procedures, p. 185. Typically F1 doctors are not required to gain patients' consent for surgery, as this should be done by the surgeon. However, the patients, who naturally have concerns regarding surgery, will ask the junior doctor about their operation. Always remember the limits of your knowledge, especially regarding the statistics of side effects: these vary with the surgical technique, as well as age, gender, etc.

A general template is:

- Introduce yourself.
- Check the patient's understanding of the situation.
- Explain the surgical procedure and who will undertake it.
- Clarify the reasons for the surgery being undertaken and its benefits.
- Inform the patient of the risks associated with the surgery.
- Explain the methodology of how this surgery will be performed, including:
  - duration of the surgery
  - any special requirements before surgery, e.g. coming in 1 or 2 days before the surgery, bowel clearout, antibiotics
  - what the surgery will entail
  - recovery pattern expected
  - follow-up advice after the surgery and post-surgery management.
- Make sure the patient understands what might happen if the surgery isn't undertaken.
- Explain alternatives to the surgery.
- Summarise and answer any questions the patient may have; offer a surgery fact sheet.

Read *Preoperation clinic*, p. 90, and consult local protocols for common medications such as aspirin and the oral contraceptive pill. This is critical for elective procedures.

EXPLAINING APPENDICECTOMY

When explaining appendicectomy to a patient admitted for appendicitis under general surgical care:

- Introduce yourself.
- Check the patient's understanding and expectations.

Surgery and reasons

You are suffering from appendicitis. We need to remove your appendix to cure your symptoms. We recommend surgery because the appendix is inflamed and there is a serious risk that it might affect the other parts of the bowel. If the appendix burst, that would lead to serious infection. These are surgical emergencies and would need immediate, complicated surgery.

Benefits

Surgery will cure your symptoms and prevent the serious complications from occurring.

Risks

The main risks are:

- *pain from the operation*
- *scarring and pain at the wound site*
- *bleeding and bruising, infection, and blood clots in the leg*
- *possible side effects from the general anaesthetic.*

Rare risks include damage to nearby structures and organs, such as the bowel – and in women the uterus, fallopian tubes and ovaries.

Methodology

Duration

The surgery will take about an hour; however, the total time may vary because of recovery time and preparation for surgery.

Preparatory work

You must stop eating and drinking from midnight before the day of the surgery. You will have lines inserted into your veins to allow us to give you fluid and anaesthetic. It is possible that you may need to have a tube passed down your throat to your stomach to remove any stomach contents. A bladder catheter may be inserted to drain urine.

Procedure

You will be seen by the anaesthetist before surgery to see how medically fit you are for surgery. You will be put to sleep by the anaesthetist, who will monitor your progress throughout the operation and in recovery. In the theatre, the surgeon will make a cut in the lower right area of the abdomen, which will serve as the entry site for removing the appendix.

After the appendix is removed, the site will be sewn up with special sutures and the skin closed. An alternative way, though not as common yet, is to remove the appendix using keyhole surgery. This would reduce scarring. The decision will be made by the surgeon at the time.

After the operation

You will be taken back to recovery and then to the ward, where the effects of the anaesthetic will wear off. All lines will be removed, including any tubes and catheters, and you will be encouraged to move around and eat and drink normally. After a few hours, and almost certainly by the next day, you will feel better and then the team will send you home. You will feel some discomfort and swelling at the wound site.

This operation generally doesn't need a consultant to follow up afterwards, so the post-operation stage will be managed by your GP. If you need antibiotics because the operation was more complex than at first thought, you will need to stay in hospital for a few days and may need antibiotics on discharge. The stitches can be removed around 10 days after the operation, and this can be done by the district nurse.

Alternatives

One possible option is to wait for the appendix to settle down by itself. However, there is an increasing risk that the appendix will become more inflamed and damage other structures. It could burst and cause inflammation to the entire tummy area. This would be life threatening and require immediate surgery.

At the end of the interview

Summarise and answer any questions the patient may have; offer a surgery fact sheet.

EXPLAINING LAPAROSCOPIC CHOLECYSTECTOMY

When explaining elective laparoscopic cholecystectomy to a patient:
- Introduce yourself.
- Check the patient's understanding and expectations.

Surgery and reasons

We would like to perform keyhole surgery to remove your gall bladder. Previously you had attacks of colicky abdominal pain, caused by your gallstones. We believe that removing the gall bladder will put an end to your symptoms.

Benefits

Removing the gall bladder will cure the symptoms you are suffering from. Keyhole surgery produces minimal scarring and has a faster recovery time than normal surgery.

Risks

With all surgery, the main problems are:

- *pain afterwards*
- *possible bleeding, bruising, swelling, infection and the risk of a blood clot in the legs*
- *the effects of the anaesthetic.*

In addition, the further risks of this particular operation are:

- *a 10% risk that the gall bladder cannot be removed using the keyhole removal technique*
- *a small risk that the gall bladder artery might be damaged, causing sudden bleeding*
- *damage to a common duct that also drains the liver*
- *a small risk of damaging local organs such as the liver and bowel.*

These complications are very rarely fatal.

If complications occur, we may need to create a larger scar beneath the rib cage to remove the gall bladder and correct any complications. You may also need intravenous antibiotics after the operation, depending on the findings. Should complications occur, you would be in hospital for around a week, compared to 1 or 2 days normally.

Other possible problems include a poor reaction to the anaesthetic, though the anaesthetist will come to see you before surgery to assess you.

Methodology

Duration

It takes around 2 hours to perform a cholecystectomy; however, it is necessary to add preparation and recovery time.

Preparatory work

You can come in the day before or on the morning of the surgery. You must not eat from midnight on the day of the surgery. Intravenous lines will be inserted for fluids and will serve as an entry point for the anaesthetic.

Procedure

You will be seen by the anaesthetist before surgery to see how medically fit you are for surgery. You will be put to sleep by the anaesthetist, who will monitor your progress throughout the operation and in recovery. You may also need to have a tube passed down your throat to your stomach to drain the contents of your stomach. You may need a bladder catheter.

The surgeon will need to make four small cuts in the abdomen, one for the camera to see inside the abdomen, and the others by which the surgeon operates the instruments. He will then remove the gall bladder. Afterwards, the surgeon will close the small holes. Quite often, an X-ray (cholangiogram) is taken during surgery of the gall bladder area – this is to look for possible remaining stones and provides an accurate record in case of future issues.

After the operation

Immediately after surgery, you will go back to the recovery room to wait for the anaesthetic to wear off. You will be monitored by the nurses and doctors.

You will then be taken back to the ward to recover. The normal stay is one night in hospital. The next day, the team will review you and probably discharge you, although this may happen on the day of the operation. All lines will be removed, including any tubes and catheters, and you will be encouraged to move around and eat and drink normally.

Depending on how complex the operation proves to be, the consultant will make a decision about whether or not they need to see you in the outpatient department. It may be that your GP can look after you. However, if there are any complications, you will need to stay in hospital longer, e.g. for antibiotics.

Alternatives

You will continue to suffer from your present symptoms if you choose not to have your gall bladder removed. Removing your gall bladder surgically is the most definitive action we can take. There are a few alternatives, such as watching and waiting; you may, for example, be symptom free for a year. There is also a chemical therapy, whereby the gallstones can be dissolved, but this is not always effective.

At the end of the interview

Summarise and answer any questions the patient may have; offer a surgery fact sheet.

EXPLAINING INGUINAL HERNIA REPAIR

A typical scenario would be explaining inguinal hernia repair to an elderly gentleman admitted for elective repair:

- Introduce yourself.
- Check the patient's understanding and expectations.

Surgery and reasons

We would like to repair your hernia, making a small cut and using a mesh to hold the hernia in place. Repairing the hernia will stop any future complications, such as the hernia becoming larger and causing a change in your bowel habit. If we don't repair the hernia, more serious complications could arise, such as the bowel twisting itself and cutting off its blood supply and dying. This would be a surgical emergency and potentially fatal.

Benefits

- *The complications detailed above will be prevented.*
- *Cosmetically the lump will be reduced.*
- *Any further lump will be prevented from developing.*
- *Pain in the groin from the hernia will usually disappear.*

Risks

Commonly, risks include pain, infection at the wound site, bleeding, bruising, swelling, scarring and blood clots in the legs. A minority of repairs fail and may require repeat surgery. For men, in rare cases, the spermatic cord and the nerves that supply the male genitals can be damaged, leading to a loss of sensation.

Methodology

Duration

The operation will take about 1 hour; however, that does not include waiting times and recovery times from surgery.

Preparatory work

You must stop eating and drinking from midnight before the day of the operation. You can take your medication if you need to. Intravenous lines will be inserted for fluids and for anaesthetic.

Procedure

You will be seen by the anaesthetist before surgery to see how medically fit you are for surgery. You will be put to sleep by the anaesthetist, who will monitor your progress throughout the operation and in recovery. You may also need to have a tube passed down your throat to your stomach to drain the contents of your stomach. You may need a bladder catheter.

The surgeon has two options: they could cut above the hernia and push the protruding tissue back into place. They would then put a mesh over the site and fix it to the local area to prevent the hernia reoccurring. A second way would be to use a camera technique (laparoscopy); in this case, they would make three suture holes: one for the camera to be inserted, and the other two for instruments to complete the operation. A mesh will also be used to secure the hernia down. They would suture your skin after removing all the equipment.

After the operation

Immediately after surgery, you will go back to the recovery room to wait for the anaesthetic to wear off. You will be monitored by the nurses and doctors.

You will then be wheeled back to the ward to recover. The normal stay is a night in hospital. The next day, the team will review you and probably discharge you, although this can happen on the day of the operation. All lines will be removed, including any tubes and catheters, and you will be encouraged to move around and eat and drink normally.

You can go home the following day – or even the same day with suitable painkillers. The local nurse will check your dressings and change them as required. If you develop an infection and need antibiotics, you may be in hospital for a longer period of time.

Alternatives

If we didn't repair the hernia, there would be a risk of complications. Apart from surgery, there are no other methods of definitively reducing the hernia. The biggest risk is that the hernia's blood supply can be cut off, which can lead to that section of the bowel dying. This is a medical emergency and would need urgent surgery. Wearing truss belts helps control the symptoms but will not correct a hernia.

At the end of the interview

- Check the patient's understanding.
- Summarise and answer any questions.
- Offer a patient leaflet about hernia surgery.

10 OSCE scenarios

This section contains some scenarios to help you to put into practice the guidance given in this book. We have not suggested what you should actually say, as your delivery should be individual to you. All scenarios are based on the chapter headings. It should be noted that in clinical practice, there could be many aspects occurring in a single scenario, such as breaking bad news, explaining a disease, and explaining management in your clinical setting.

You might like to get a small group of fellow students together to practise. We have provided roles for both the doctor and the patient to reflect real-life situations and make the practice more realistic.

At the end of each scenario, we have listed the key communication and legal issues.

SCENARIO 1 – NEW DIAGNOSIS OF ASTHMA

Doctor role

You are a foundation year-one doctor in the clinic with your consultant. Please explain to Johnny, a 15-year-old school boy, a new diagnosis of asthma. He was admitted last month for severe dyspnoea and wheeze over the preceding 2 weeks. He recently had his spirometry assessment, which showed a reversible obstructive lung defect. He does not know his diagnosis. You do not need to explain medication or inhalers, since the asthma nurse will later be spending time with him and his mother.

Patient role

You are Johnny, a 15-year-old boy. You have come to the clinic today and are rather frightened about what happened to you last month. You are attending with your mother and are embarrassed by that fact. You were secretly hoping you could have left home already. You have no idea what the doctor will tell you, but are willing to listen.

Key issues that need to be addressed

- Breaking bad news, p. 24
- Explaining diseases, p. 107
- Legal consent and the issues regarding parent and child, p. 37
- This scenario could be expanded to include explaining asthma medication, p. 152.

SCENARIO 2 – EXPLAINING ASTHMA MEDICATION

Doctor role

The asthma nurse is away on annual leave and you have been asked to provide emergency cover for her. Johnny, the patient from Scenario 1, is your next patient. You have been asked to explain the value of salbutamol and beclometasone to him. Please explain to Johnny what his medication is for and how to use his inhalers.

Patient role

You are Johnny, the 15-year-old boy from Scenario 1. You have had a bad encounter with this doctor previously and you are shocked that the same doctor is now going to tell you 'how to live your life'. Play the role of the troublesome teenager.

Key issues that need to be addressed

- Explaining drugs and medication, p. 152
- Explaining devices, p. 175

- Dealing with difficult patients, p. 49. You must be able to demonstrate empathy towards the (adolescent) patient
- Legal status of children and young people, p. 37.

Refer to: Explaining asthma, p. 108; Explaining asthma medication, p. 152; Explaining inhalers, p. 177; Explaining peak flow meters, p. 175.

SCENARIO 3 – COMBINED ORAL CONTRACEPTIVE PILL

Doctor role

You are a registrar on the GP training programme. You have to see Lisa, a 15-year-old girl, who is accompanied by her anxious mother. The daughter asks to see you alone, a request which you and the mother agree to. During the consultation, Lisa asks you about the availability of the oral contraceptive pill, because, unknown to her mother, she has been seeing an 18-year-old boy for the past 6 months, and she is ready to have sex with him.

Patient role

You are Lisa, a 15-year-old girl. You have been going steady with your 18-year-old boyfriend for 6 months and you are ready to have sex with him. You know that if your mother found out she would be very angry and prevent you from seeing him. But you are sensible enough to think about avoiding pregnancy, as a girl in your year at school had to leave for maternity reasons.

Mother's role

You are Lisa's mother, and are a bit upset that your daughter has asked you not to attend her consultation. After the consultation, you approach the doctor, shouting and demanding to know what was discussed. You think the consultation was about drugs or sex.

Key issues that need to be addressed

- Legal nature of the medical interview with a child under 16 years old, p. 36; also ethical considerations about informing the mother.
- Taking a sexual history, p. 72.
- Explaining the oral contraceptive pill, p. 159.

Refer to Gillick competence, p. 39.

SCENARIO 4 – HIV TEST COUNSELLING

Doctor role

A patient, who was admitted whilst your firm was on take yesterday, has a plethora of mismatched symptoms. He has disclosed that, 6 months ago, one of his lovers was HIV positive. With HIV a strong possibility now, as the foundation year-one (F1) doctor, you've been asked by your consultant to counsel this patient for an HIV test and determine his HIV status. Unfortunately, the nearest sexual clinic is 10 miles away, and the patient has already stated that, because of the distance, he does not want to go there.

Patient role

You are a 25-year-old man, and have come in because of unexplained rashes, fevers, lumps in your groin and bruising. On the ward round, when asked, you admitted that your ex-boyfriend was found to be HIV positive around 6 months ago. You were contact traced and have not had the time to be tested. Also, because of your fears of the possible diagnosis, you have not been inclined to undergo the test. The consultant has explained that one of the team will come back later in the day to counsel you for HIV testing. You have agreed in principle to this, but you want to know when the results would come back and how you should pick them up.

Key issues that need to be addressed

- Determining level of risk of HIV infection.
- Pre-HIV test counselling, p. 100, especially disclosing results.
- Taking a sexual history, p. 72.
- Legal status of HIV, p. 102.

SCENARIO 5 – HIV TEST RESULTS COUNSELLING

Doctor role

You are the F1 doctor from Scenario 4, who took the blood sample for the HIV test for this patient. You explained to the patient the need to come back in 1 week's time to the ward to get his results. He has arrived and he is drinking a cup of tea in the relatives' room. You look up his result and it is HIV positive. Before you see him, you briefly talk to your registrar to get the facts and figures correct before you proceed.

Patient role

You have come back for the results with great dread. You feel ill at the thought of the possible outcome of the test. When told it is positive, you do not know how to readjust your life and you break down and cry. You can't cope with what the doctor is saying and eventually you leave the room.

Key issues that need to be addressed

- Breaking bad news, p. 24
- Explaining an HIV-positive result, p. 101
- Legal status of HIV, p. 102.

SCENARIO 6 – LAPAROSCOPIC CHOLECYSTECTOMY

Doctor role

You are a foundation year-two (F2) doctor on your surgical rotation. You have been asked to obtain consent, provisionally, from a middle-aged lady who has come in for a laparoscopic cholecystectomy. Your consultant will shortly be up to review what you have told her, but he wants you to start first. You find that her English is not very good.

Patient role

You are a middle-aged lady, who has been getting attacks of upper abdominal pain for the past year since coming to the UK from India. When you were admitted 6 months ago, an ultrasound revealed that you had gallstones. About 2 months ago the consultant discussed the benefits of an operation to remove the gallbladder, but because it was so long ago you don't remember what he said. You are worried about the operation, since an operation 25 years ago to remove your appendix resulted in a week's stay in hospital, with you needing antibiotics.

Key issues that need to be addressed

- Consenting for the operation, p. 11.
- Explaining the risks and benefits appropriately.

- Legal issues if the patient does not speak English, p. 43

Refer to Explaining laparoscopic cholecystectomy, p. 216.

SCENARIO 7 – ANGINA PATIENT

Doctor role

You are a foundation year-one (F1) doctor, who is helping out in the consultant clinic. You have been passed a set of notes about a patient who was admitted for chest pain, which turned out to be angina. The patient also has a history of hypertension, and their medication was changed to lisinopril because of the side effects of atenolol. You have been asked to assess how he is. As the patient walks in, you are bombarded with a list of questions about what angina is and the link between high blood pressure and angina. The patient has not taken any of his pills or the GTN spray.

Patient role

You are a patient who is angry because of the lack of explanation given for your condition. On your last admission, you were originally told that the diagnosis was inflammation of the sac of fluid around the heart. However, on discharge you were told that you had angina. The nurses gave you your bag of medication and said that your appointment with the doctor would be sent in the post. That is all that you have heard from the hospital and you have had difficulty getting any further information from your GP.

Key issues that need to be addressed

- Poor adherence to medication, p. 52.
- Dealing with the angry patient, p. 49.

- Explaining atenolol/GTN spray, p. 146.
- Explaining angina, p. 114.
- Legal status of the competent adult, p. 11.

SCENARIO 8 – DEPRESSION, ANXIETY AND SUICIDE

Doctor role

You are a final-year medical student, on the last day of your finals. Your final station is to take a history from a 25-year-old man. He was brought into the emergency department, having been found unconscious in his flat earlier today by his girlfriend, with an empty bottle of lorazepam tablets and some tequila. The psychiatric team are going to send him home today, with follow-up in 2 months. A prescription for fluoxetine has been given to continue after he goes home.

Patient role

You are a 25-year-old US investment banker who, 1 month ago, was sacked after an investigation at your bank revealed your insider trading. As a result, you may be barred from working in banking ever again and deported back to the US to face criminal charges. It was a great shock when you were sacked this morning, and you broke down at your flat. You took the whole bottle of your girlfriend's sleeping tablets (around 30) and drank a bottle of tequila over a few hours. You don't remember passing out, but the next thing you remember is your girlfriend crying and trying to wake you up. After that, you remember waking up in hospital. This act was impulsive, but you had been feeling suicidal for the past month.

A medical student wants to interview you, but you are in no mood to talk. However, after some persistence, you begin answering the student's questions. You ask him about depression and how it can be managed, and whether medication will help.

Key issues that need to be addressed

- Psychiatric history and mental health, p. 78.
- Suicide history.
- Explaining depression, p. 111 and Explaining SSRI drugs, p. 150.
- Legal: Mental Capacity Act, p. 11 and mental illness.

1 Appendix 1 – Clinical negligence

WHEN A PATIENT SUES

If a patient is to successfully sue a doctor, they must prove that:

1. the doctor owed them a duty of care;
2. the doctor breached that duty;
3. as a result of that breach, they suffered loss;
4. the loss suffered is of a type compensatable by the court.

THE DUTY OF CARE

A doctor owes a duty of care to his patients in the ordinary course of events.

THE HEALTH AUTHORITY/TRUST

A Health Authority/Trust has a duty to provide services of health professionals of sufficient skill and is therefore liable for any failure to provide such services.

BREACH OF THE DUTY OF CARE

In order to show a breach of duty of care, the patient must prove that the doctor's actions are not supported by any responsible body of medical opinion. This is the Bolam test.

The starting point in Scotland is the test set out in *Hunter v Hanley* (1955) where, to establish liability, the Court of Session required three elements to be established:

1. There is a usual and normal practice.
2. The defender has not adopted that practice.
3. The course adopted by the defender was one which no professional man of ordinary skill would have adopted.

The facts of the Bolam case

John Bolam was admitted to Friern Mental Hospital in 1954, suffering from depression. He was treated with electroconvulsive therapy (ECT). If no relaxant drug is administered, one of the effects of ECT is to cause fits, muscular contractions and spasms carrying a slight risk of bone fracture. Mr Bolam was not warned by the hospital of the risks of the ECT treatment. He underwent ECT without a relaxant drug being administered and without being given any form of manual restraint, and he sustained hip fractures.

Mr Bolam alleged that the hospital was negligent in failing to administer him a suitable relaxant drug before the ECT, failing to provide manual control whilst he was fitting, and failing to warn him of the risks of ECT. *Bolam v Friern Hospital Management Committee* [1957] 1 WLR 583.

The Bolam test has been developed by the case of *Bolitho v City and Hackney Health Authority* [1998] AC 232 (HL).

The facts of the Bolitho case

Patrick Bolitho was diagnosed with acute croup in January 1984 and admitted to St Bartholomew's Hospital.

At 12.40 p.m. on 17 January 1984, the ward sister found that Patrick's respiratory sounds were poor and he was white in colour. The sister bleeped the Paediatric Senior Registrar, who said that she would attend Patrick as soon as possible. Patrick improved, but at around 2.00 p.m., after a similar episode, the ward sister telephoned the senior registrar again, as she had not yet attended. The senior registrar attempted to ask the senior house officer to attend in her place. However, the SHO's bleep was not working and she did not receive the message. At about 2.35 p.m. Patrick collapsed, unable to breathe, and suffered a cardiac arrest and severe brain damage.

> Bolitho developed the 'Bolam' test by insisting that, even if a doctor can say they acted in accordance with a reasonable body of medical opinion, that opinion must still be able to withstand logical analysis.

If it can be shown that the doctor acted in accordance with a *'responsible, reasonable and logical body of opinion'*, there will be a defence to the action. The test is objective and inexperience is no defence. The courts have acknowledged that, in the realms of diagnosis and treatment, there is plenty of scope for differences of opinion and a doctor should not be deemed negligent simply because his opinion differs from that of other doctors. A specialist is expected to achieve the standard of care of the reasonably competent specialist practising in that field. The more skilled a doctor is, the higher the standard expected of them.

The burden of proof is on the patient to show that, on the balance of probability, there was a breach of duty. Remember that just because a procedure goes wrong, it does not necessarily mean that there has been a breach of duty.

BREACH CAUSING HARM

The patient will have to show that, 'but for' the negligent treatment by the doctor, they would have recovered (either fully or partly) from their pre-existing condition. Alternatively, they will maintain that their condition was made worse or that injuries unconnected with their condition were caused.

A claimant does not receive damages for lost chances of recovery if they were less than 50% in any event. The test criterion is: 'but for' the negligence, the patient would not, on a balance of probability, have suffered the harm in any event.

COMPENSATABLE LOSS

Patients must show that they experienced a reasonable fore-seeable loss. If they are able to do so, they will be compensated in the form of damages, i.e. money.

General damages and special damages

General damages compensate for pain and suffering, whereas special damages compensate for past and future pecuniary loss. The aim of damages is to restore the patient to the position they were in before the incident.

2 Appendix 2 – A summary of British legal structure

CIVIL COURTS

People or organisations resolve their disputes in the Civil Court. Usually one party is suing another for money to compensate them, for example for injuries allegedly caused by the negligence of the other party.

Examples of Civil Courts in England and Wales: County Courts; the High Court.

Examples of Civil Courts in Scotland: the Sheriff Court; the Court of Session.

The burden and standard of proof

The **burden of proof** is usually carried by the party bringing the case, i.e. the Claimant.

The **standard of proof** is the degree to which a case must be proved by the party with the burden of proof.

In the Civil Courts the standard of proof is **on the balance of probability**, or to put it another way, is something **more likely than not**.

FAMILY COURTS

Special Family Courts hear divorce and child contact cases. These courts also deal with child protection cases, which are brought by local authorities. These courts only sit in England

and Wales. Family cases come before the ordinary Civil Courts in Scotland, although they proceed under special rules.

Examples of Family Courts in England and Wales:
- Family Proceedings Court
- Care Centres
- The Principal Registry of the Family Division (in London)
- High Court.

The burden and standard of proof

The burden of proof is usually carried by the party bringing the case, i.e. the Applicant.

The standard of proof is on the balance of probability.

CRIMINAL COURTS

When the Crown prosecutes an individual or organisation, the matter is heard in the Criminal Courts.

Examples of Criminal Courts in England and Wales:
- The Magistrates' Court
- Crown Court
- Old Bailey
- Central Criminal Court (in London).

Examples of Criminal Courts in Scotland:
- District Court
- Sheriff Court
- High Court of Justiciary in Scotland.

The burden and standard of proof

The burden of proof is usually on the Crown.

The standard of proof is beyond a reasonable doubt, or to put it another way, the Court must be sure.

REGULATORY FORUMS

These are hearings conducted by professional bodies, during which individual practitioners answer allegations about their practice. They generally have jurisdiction throughout Great Britain.

Examples of Regulatory Forums:
- General Medical Council (GMC)
- Nursing and Midwifery Council (NMC)
- Health Professions Council (HPC) Fitness to Practise hearings.

The burden and standard of proof

The burden of proof is usually on the party bringing the case, namely the Fitness to Practise panel for the GMC.

Cases are decided before the GMC Fitness to Practise Panel using the civil standard of proof (on the balance of probability).

EMPLOYMENT TRIBUNALS

Employment Tribunals are forums where disputes relating to employment rights are decided.

The burden and standard of proof

The party bringing the case, namely the employee, will usually carry the burden of proof.

Cases are decided using the civil standard of proof (on the balance of probability).

CORONER'S COURTS

A Coroner's Court is a forum for examining the circumstances surrounding a violent, unnatural or sudden death where the cause of death is unclear, occurs in a hospital or is otherwise required by law.

The Coroner conducts, with or without a jury, a fact-finding inquiry to establish answers to the following questions:

- Who died?
- Where did they die?
- When did they die?
- How did they die, i.e. what was the mechanism by which they met their death?

In theory, an inquest does not apportion blame. However, there is the possible (though rare) verdict of **neglect**.

There is also the new **narrative** verdict. The narrative verdict is now common and indicates that a death took place for a series of reasons. Whilst a verdict of this type does not apportion blame, it can paint the circumstances of a death in a very unflattering light.

The Coroner can, on the basis of their findings, make recommendations with regard to institutions.

Cases are decided (with the exception of those involving suicide) on a balance of probability.

In Scotland, deaths of the kind described above must be reported to the Procurator Fiscal. When a Fatal Accident Inquiry is heard, the role of the Coroner's Court is fulfilled by the Sheriff Court. The procedure is broadly similar to that adopted by the Coroner's Court.

3 Appendix 3 – Notifiable diseases

NOTIFIABLE DISEASES

- Acute encephalitis
- Acute poliomyelitis
- Anthrax
- Cholera
- Diphtheria
- Dysentery
- Food poisoning
- Leptospirosis
- Malaria
- Measles
- Meningitis
- Meningococcal septicaemia (without meningitis)
- Mumps
- Ophthalmia neonatorum
- Paratyphoid fever
- Plague
- Rabies
- Relapsing fever
- Rubella
- Scarlet fever
- Smallpox
- Tetanus
- Tuberculosis
- Typhoid fever
- Typhus fever

- Viral haemorrhagic fever
- Viral hepatitis
- Whooping cough
- Yellow fever

Leprosy is also notifiable, but directly to the Health Protection Agency (HPA) and the Centre for Infection (CFI).

Index

C

D